MINIINVASIVE TECHNIQUES IN RHINOPLASTY

Edited by **Nikolay Serdev**

Miniinvasive Techniques in Rhinoplasty
http://dx.doi.org/10.5772/60908
Edited by Nikolay Serdev

Contributors

Nikolay Serdev

Published by InTech

Janeza Trdine 9, 51000 Rijeka, Croatia

Publishing Process Manager Danijela Duric

Technical Editor InTech DTP team

Cover InTech Design team

First published March, 2016

Printed in Croatia

Additional hard copies can be obtained from orders@intechopen.com

Miniinvasive Techniques in Rhinoplasty, Edited by Nikolay Serdev

p. cm.

ISBN 978-953-51-2260-9

For EU product safety concerns:
IN TECH d.o.o., Prolaz Marije Krucifikse Kozulić 3, 51000 Rijeka, Croatia,
info@intechopen.com or visit our website at intechopen.com.

Meet the editor

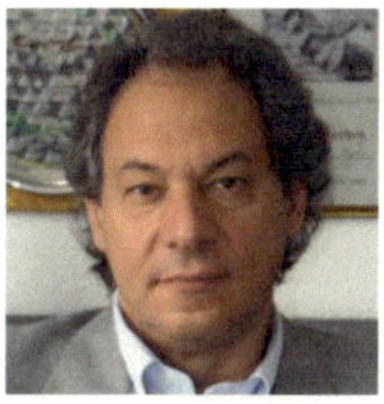

Prof. Dr. Nikolay Serdev, MD, PhD is a renowned cosmetic doctor and surgeon. He has trained hundreds of doctors globally, in minimally invasive aesthetic surgery and medical procedures. He is a founding member of the European Society of Aesthetic Surgery and the International Board of Cosmetic Surgery. He is a Honorary President of the Bulgarian Society of Aesthetic Surgery and Aesthetic Medicine, Honorary Professor of the New Bulgarian University, the International College of Cosmetic Surgery, the South East Asia College of Cosmet - ic Surgery, Honorary member of the Australian College of Cosmetic Surgery, South American Academy of Cosmetic Surgery, French Society of Aesthetic Surgery and numerous other international societies. Dr. Serdev is the author of "Scarless Serdev Suture® lifts" of face and body and pioneer in many mini-invasive cosmetic surgery techniques: ultrasound liposculpture of face, body; leg elongation and beautifica - tion; T-excision and columella sliding in rhinoplasty; non-surgical body contouring; and combination approaches to facial volumising and rejuvenation. He is also a world authority in ultrasound-assisted (VASER) body contouring and has trained doctors from around the world in its basic and advanced techniques. Dr. Serdev divides his time between his clinic, the New Bulgarian University in Sofia and short travels for hands-on courses in countries of all continents. He is editor of the most comprehen - sive textbook in Liposuction and has authored many chapters in aesthetic surgery and medicine, as well as original papers in leading medical journals.

Contents

Preface

Facial harmony and aesthetics often depend on small individual characteristics in proportions, volumes and angles, requiring understanding of art and perfection in treatment, which is critical in rhinoplasty. It is an artistic procedure to give the highly demanded proportions and angles, as well as properly localized volumes as an aesthetic part of the whole face, which is the goal of beautification. Patient's age, sex, skin quality, ethnicity should be considered. Nasal tip position has great importance in all cases of rhinoplasty and especially in cases of long, short or non-proportional noses.

Over the past decades surgical and medical techniques have greatly progressed to improve and correct appearance and breathing. In recent years, due to the dynamic modern lifestyle, there is diminishing in numbers of extended traumatic rhinoplasty operations. Many mini-invasive surgical and non-surgical techniques were introduced to be more atraumatic and to prevent cartilages from iatrogenic trauma and devascularization, thus permitting faster healing and a more stable result.

There is an increasing patient and doctor interest in procedures without trauma or scars. Prolonged surgery, downtime, and absence from work and social life have provoked a notable development in mini-invasive techniques. Nowadays minimally invasive surgical and non-surgical procedures have been indicated and available for the treatment of asymmetries, smaller irregularities, post-surgical defects and even airflow problems. In many primary and secondary cases, aesthetic problems exist, which do not need an open rhinoplasty and the full armament of bone-cartilage treatment that can be more traumatic than necessary.

Dr Nikolay Serdev, MD, PhD
Medical Center "Aesthetic Surgery, Aesthetic Medicine"
Bulgaria

Section 1

Surgical Techniques

Chapter 1

T-Excision for Nasal Tip Rotation

Nikolay P. Serdev

Additional information is available at the end of the chapter

http://dx.doi.org/10.5772/62061

Abstract

Authors "T-excision" for nasal tip rotation is used to reduce long noses as an independent procedure or as a part of primary or secondary rhinoplasties. It consists of "en bloc" excision of the cephalic part of the greater alar cartilages and elongated caudal septum, using: 1) total retrocolumellar incision, prolonged in transcartilaginous incisions, through opposite nostrils, leaving only skin intact; 2) septal incision, perpendicular to dorsum to form correct dorsum length, prolonged into intercartilaginous incisions, through opposite nostrils, leaving only skin intact. Thus, the cephalic strip resection is done en bloc with the unnecessary excessive and prolonged septum and soft tissue. Two, three mattress transmucosal septocolumellar sutures for 2–3 weeks are enough to support healing. The T-excision technique is mini-invasive, nearly bloodless, and time-saving. It is safe; well-tolerated by patients; there is no pain after surgery; no need of plaster, tampons, and bandages. Patients can return next day to social life and work.

Keywords: Rhinoplasty, long nose, T-excision en bloc, mini-invasive technique, elongated septum, primary or secondary, retrocolumellar incision, transcartilaginous incision, intercartilaginous incisions, perpendicular to dorsum septal incision, no downtime

1. Introduction

Facial analysis is critical in rhinoplasty. This procedure is not an operation of a separated nose; it is an artistic surgery to give aesthetic proportions and angles, as well as properly localized volumes as an aesthetic part of the whole face, which is the goal of beautification. Patient's age, sex, skin quality, ethnicity should be considered. Nasal tip position has great importance in all cases of rhinoplasty and especially in cases of long and nonproportional nose. Cephalic strip resection of the lower lateral cartilages is performed to achieve upward tip rotation. The "en bloc" T-excision technique for adjustment of nasal tip involves new understanding of well-known incisions, based on anatomical knowledge and specific surgical skills. It minimizes trauma, it is nearly bloodless, achieving acceptable beautifying postoperative result with no downtime for the patient, requiring no plaster, no tampons, and nearly immediate return to work and social life. This technique prevents cartilages from iatrogenic trauma and devascularization and thus permits faster healing and a stable result. It includes cephalic strip resection and septal shortening (caudal septum and/or retrocolumellar mucosal elongation) en bloc.

2. Anatomy

The **greater alar cartilages** (**lower lateral cartilages**) are situated below the upper lateral nasal cartilages, forming the columella and the wings of the nostrils. The medial crura are loosely connected with the corresponding portion of the opposite cartilage. Together with the septum they stabilize the columella. In Caucasians, the columella is stable, unlike Asians, Afro-Americans, and Latino-Americans.

The author's observations in Caucasian, Asian, and Afro-American noses show that the proper dorsocolumellar angle is very near to 90^0. Angles different from the right angle change the aesthetic proportions and disbalance the beauty triangle [1-9].

3. Tip rotation

Using the tripod concept, a long nose has longer superior legs (lateral crura of greater alar cartilages) and shorter central leg (medial crura and columella). Thus, the shortening of the lateral crura (cephalic strip resection of the lower lateral cartilages) gives upward tip rotation. (**NB**: Projection of the nasal tip is described by the author in the chapter, "Columella Sliding for Nasal Tip Projection.")

Tip rotation is also related to "position of the tip to the alar crease." The angle at the nasal tip has been described as the wide angle between the vertical line passing through the alar crease and a second line that is drawn from the alar crease to the nasal tip, on lateral view. The ideal tip angle is described to be 105º in females and 100º in males [7-9].

The author's opinion is that such description can hardly guide a surgeon during the process of operation. His observation is that angles that are too different from the right angle at the nasal tip disrupt the aesthetic proportions and the "beauty triangle" composed of both cheeks and chin (Figures 17, -11). If the angle is more acute, the nose appears to be long and disproportional to the whole face, and the nasal tip (when seen enface) hangs into the area of the upper lip. If the tip angle is obtuse, the nose appears short and over-rotated, as in some Asian and Afro-American noses.

4. Patient consent

If the tip angle is correct, the nostrils in enface aspect are slightly visible. Usually, patients with long noses, who have never seen their nostrils, have difficulty in accepting that nostrils should be a bit visible in frontal aspect. It should be clearly explained that in order for the nostrils to be invisible, the tip angle should be sharp (about 70^0), which is not appropriate and the nose looks long in relation to the face (Figure 1). Patients should be informed, confident, and motivated for this change.

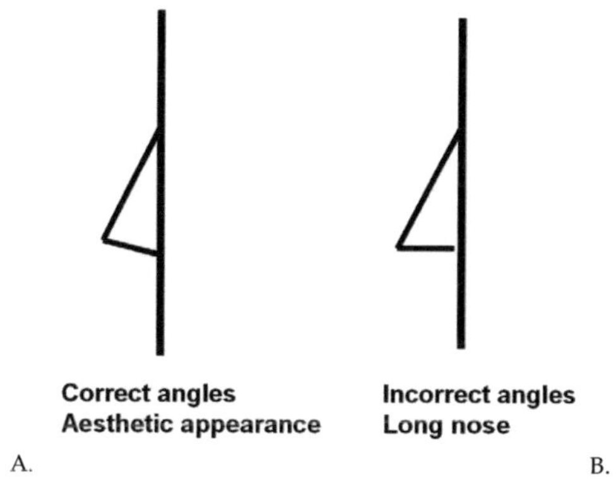

Figure 1. A. Correct aesthetic proportions and angles. The nose is proportional – 1/3 of the face. Correct 30^0 dorsoprofile angle and nasal tip angles. Nostrils should be a bit visible from a frontal view. **B.** Visibly incorrect length, angles, and lack of aesthetic section of nose and face. The nostrils are not visible from a frontal view. Long nose.

4.1. Design of the T-excision technique

Excision of the cephalic part of the **greater alar cartilages,** including unnecessary prominent caudal part of septum, permits rotation of the tip, i.e., shortening the length of the nose. The T-excision technique described below is made en bloc, using a closed rhinoplasty approach.

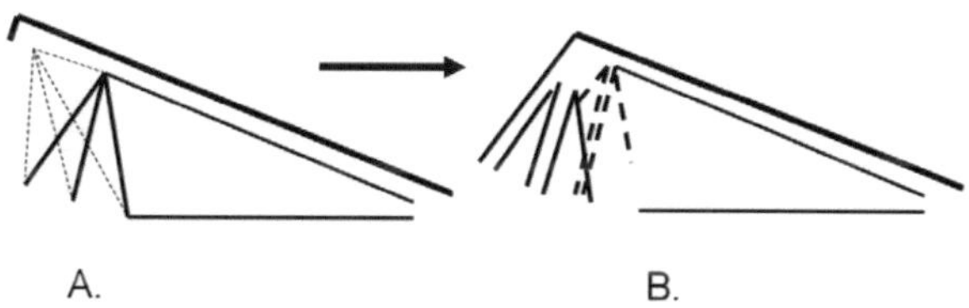

Figure 2. T-excision drawing. A. Schematic excision of 3 triangles – 2 lateral triangle excisions and one medial triangle excision perpendicular to the nasal dorsum. **B.** Result after tip rotation gives correct tip position and angles.

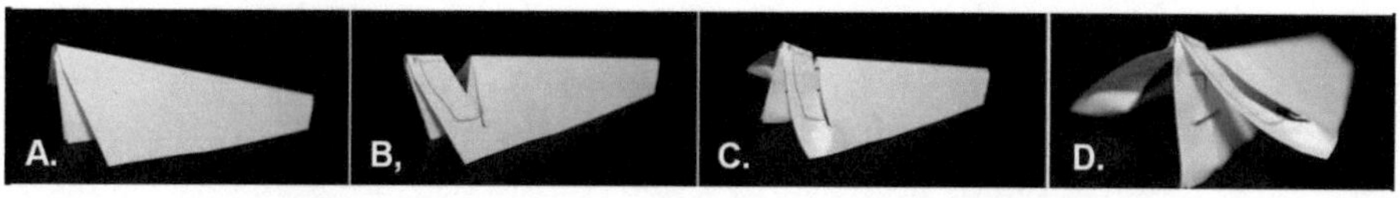

Figure 3. A. Schematic pyramid in a long nose. **B.** T-excision en bloc, including cephalic part of the greater alar cartilages and elongated caudal septum. **C.** Tip of the nose rotates easily. **D.** Two to three transmucosal mattress sutures of columella to caudal septum are enough to hold the tip in position and guarantee good fixation for healing. Stitches are removed after 2–3 weeks.

5. T-excision: Surgical technique

The initial local infiltration of anesthesia should not deform the nasal tip.

5.1. First incision

A total retrocolumellar incision is performed to separate the columella from the septum. In cases of dropping columella, this incision should follow a desired design. To remove dropping columella, the incision should leave an equal thickness along the length of the columella. Any other form should be previously designed according to patient's desire and informed consent. The **retrocolumellar incision** is then **prolonged into transcartilaginous incision**, which separates the lateral wing of the greater alar cartilage in cephalic and distal parts. In the past, the author used methylene blue dye to mark the transcartilaginous incision, but it is not always easy to exactly reflect the line that has been drawn on the external skin. Actually, this is not totally necessary, because the transcartilaginous incision is a prolongation of the retrocolumellar incision in each nostril, parallel to the nostril border. The transcartilaginous incision is performed in each nostril through the opposite nostril, using the opening of the retrocolumellar incision – this gives better visibility to the surgeon and permits for better orientation. This incision cuts mucosa and cartilages, leaving the skin intact. To be precise, both alae nasi are held with thumb and index of the other hand, feeling the scalpel below the skin with the fingertips. Transcartilaginous incisions should be located 4–5 mm cephalic to the caudal margin of the lateral crus of the lower cartilages. Finishing both transcartilaginous incisions and leaving only the skin intact, one has separated the lateral wings of the greater alar cartilage in cephalic and distal parts, whereupon the cephalic parts will be removed with the T-excision en bloc.

5.2. Second incision

The reduction of the length of the nose in the caudal septum region is selective. The second incision line is a **"90°-to-dorsum" septal incision**, starting from a selected dorsum point in a downward direction, perpendicular to the nasal dorsum to meet the retrocolumellar incision (forming the medial excision triangle), which usually happens above the nasal spine. This incision is total, including caudal septum and both sides of mucosa at once (or, in many cases, only elongated mucosa). The "90°-to-dorsum" septal incision is then prolonged into intercartilaginous incisions in both nostrils, each one through the opposite nostril using the opening of the "90°-to-dorsum" septal incision. The intercartilaginous incision should be placed minimum 2 mm caudal to the valve on the lateral crura side, in order to prevent nasal valve stenosis. The intercartilaginous incision in this technique leaves intact only the skin under the fingertips of the guiding hand, as described above. Intercartilaginous incisions meet the transcartilaginous incisions laterally, forming the 2 lateral triangles of the T-excision. Thus, cephalic parts of greater alar cartilages are separated together with the unnecessary elongated septum (or only mucosa), forming 3 triangles of the "T-excision en bloc": two lateral triangles in the nostrils and one medial triangle in the septal retrocolumellar part. The tissue of the "T-excision en bloc" is still fixed to the alar skin from which it will be separated and removed by using blunt tip scissors, guided by the other hand to prevent the alar skin from trauma.

The surrounding skin is slightly undermined with the scissors in 2–3 mm distance to permit rotation of the nasal tip and skin adaptation.

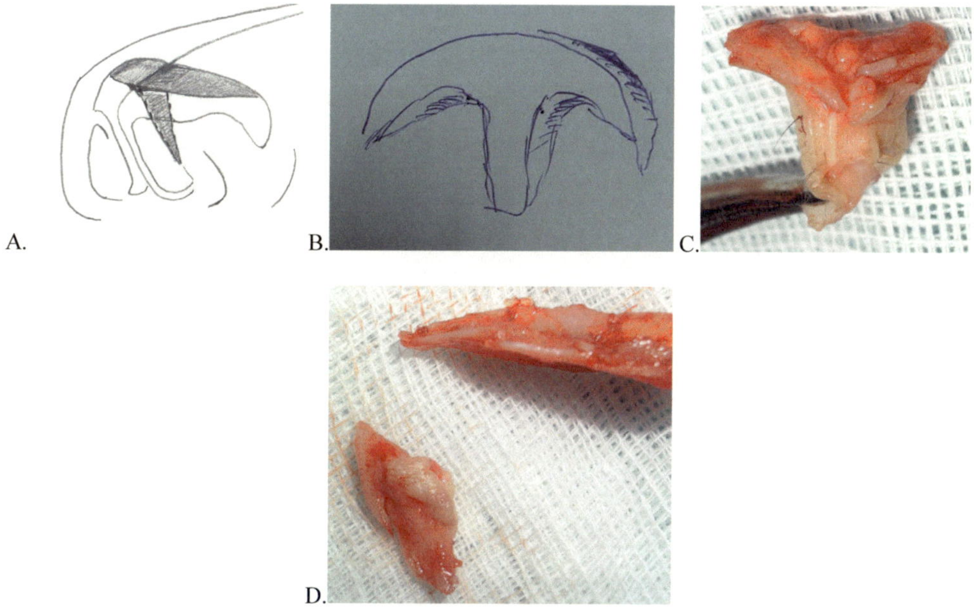

Figure 4. T-excision en bloc of 3 triangles: **A.** Transcartilaginous and intercartilaginous incisions form the 2 lateral triangles of the T-excision. The retrocolumellar and the "90°-to-dorsum" septal incision form the medial triangle of caudal septum excision. The 2 lateral triangles should include the cephalic strip of greater alar cartilages. **B.** Scheme of excised tissue. **C.** Excised T-formation en bloc. This particular T-excision en bloc includes caudal septum in the medial triangle and cephalic part of the greater alar cartilages in the lateral triangles. **D.** Humpectomy and T-excision will give the new profile form of the nose.

T-excision could be used separately in long noses, or as a part of rhinoplasty with hump removal and other additional techniques. The operation is ambulatory, under local anesthesia. The author uses additional IV sedation. The procedure is almost bloodless and atraumatic. Two to three transmucosal mattress sutures are used to fix columella to septum. Stitches are removed after 2–3 weeks, if not absorbed. There is no need of any bandages or tampons. Patients return to their social life almost immediately.

In aesthetics, there is another important aspect – the "beauty triangle," forming the mid and lower face beauty. It includes the two cheekbones and the chin. The tip of the nose should not disrupt the upper line of the triangle connecting the projection of the two cheekbones, i.e., its prominence has to be on the line between the two cheekbones. Thus, the nasal tip presents an important aesthetic facial volume, forming a straight line together with the volume of the cheekbones (Figure 7).

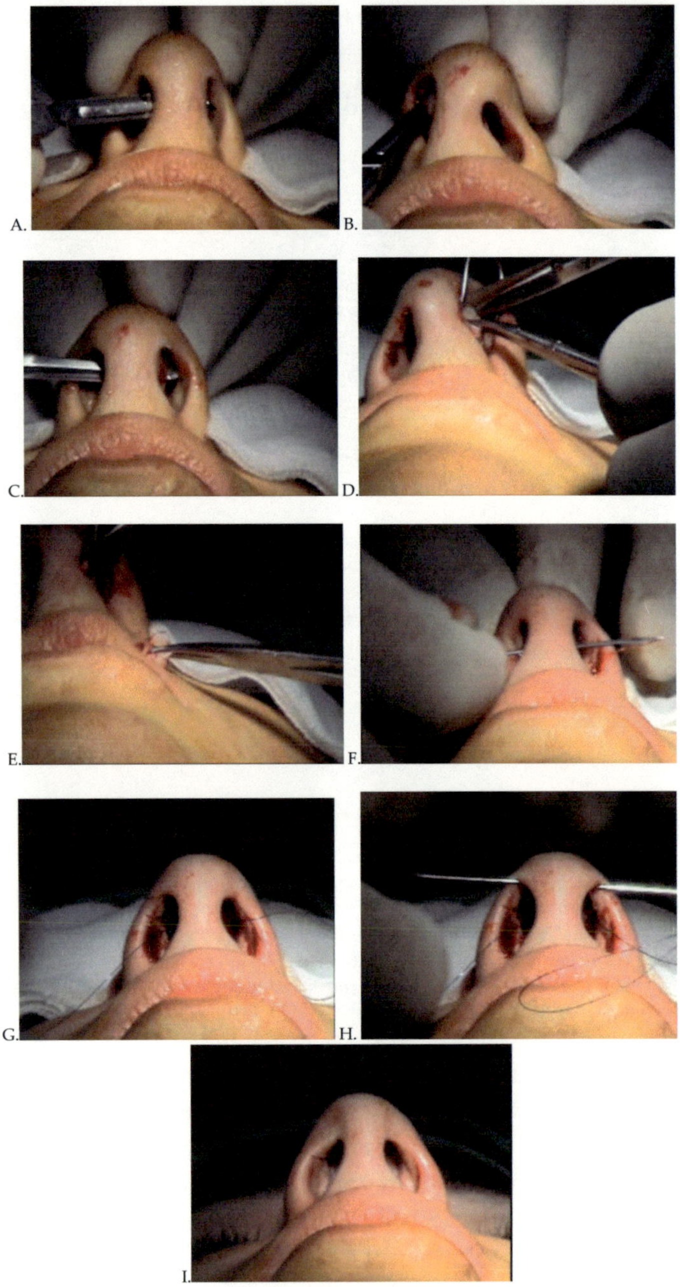

Figure 5. A. Total retrocolumellar incision. **B.** The retrocolumellar incision is prolonged into intercartilaginous incisions both sides through the opposite nostril, using the opening of the retrocolumellar incision. **C.** Second septal perpendicular to dorsum incision. It will be prolonged into 2 intercartilaginous incisions. **D.** The T-Excision en bloc is separated from the dorsal skin with a blunt tip scissor. **E** The T-excision is separated and removed, **F.** The transmucosal mattress suture is performed horizontally if the dome is symmetric (or parallel to the asymmetry). **G.** The transmucosal septocolumellar suture is ready to be knotted. **H.** Transmucosal domal suture of medial crura for tip refinement. **I.** Result after atraumatic, nearly bloodless T-excision procedure for nasal tip rotation.

http://dx.doi.org/10.5772/62061

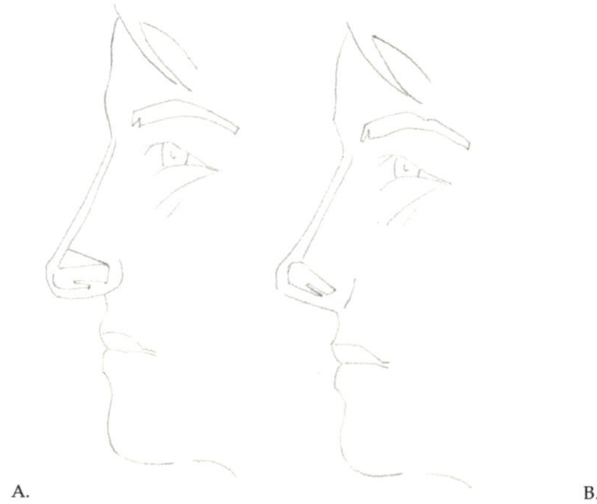

Figure 6. A. The unnecessary length of septum will be resected. B. The nasal tip is rotated and a correct tip angle is obtained, adapting the nose into 1/3 of the length of the face.

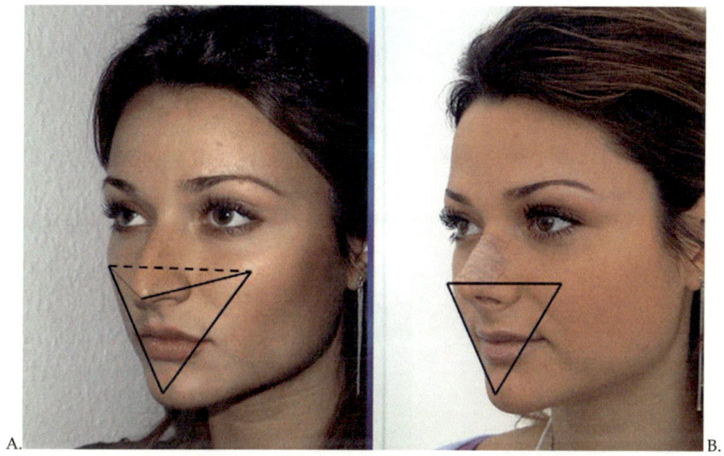

Figure 7. A case of a long nose. A. Before. The long nose causes incorrect facial proportions. The beauty triangle is disrupted, forming 2 incorrect triangles. The facial features of the patient's face are nice but nearly invisible because of the long and disproportional nose. B. After T-excision for nasal tip rotation and columella sliding for tip projection. The nose is shortened to fit into 1/3 of the face. Correct aesthetic proportions (three equal parts of the face), correct 30^0 dorsoprofile angle, and nasal tip volume on the line of the cheekbone prominence. The tape is not necessary – it was requested by the patient (a ballerina) to make the operation visible and thus protect her from trauma at work. The result is beautification of the face by correct proportions and angles and visible beauty triangle.

6. Clinical cases

Immediately after operation, local anesthesia and postoperative edema raise the dorsum and make the nasolabial angle obtuse, which gives an impression of over-rotation of the nasal tip.

It is a false impression. With the diminishing of the edema in the first 5–7 days, the correct angle takes shape and the tip falls into place.

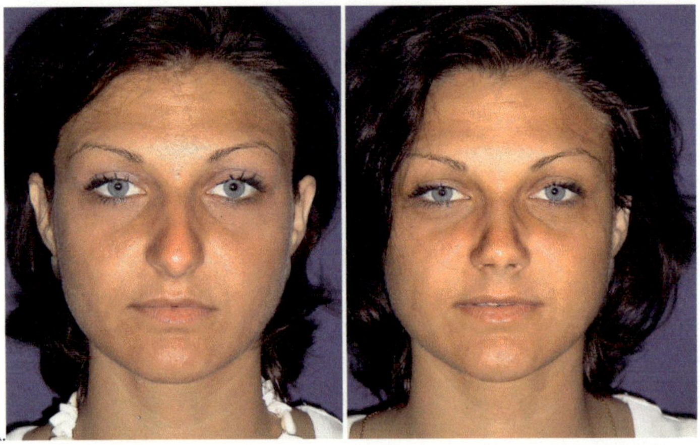

A. B.

Figure 8. T-excision for nasal tip rotation. Immediate result in a case of a long and disproportional nose. **A.** Before. Long nose with hanging columella, resulting in a disproportional face, containing some nice features, nearly invisible to observers. **B.** After. Immediate result, a few minutes after T-excision, nasal tip and lower third refinement by transcutaneous Serdev Sutures®. Swelling could be visible to specialists but not to the public. Aesthetic proportions (three equal parts of the face) are present. The result is beautification of the face – previously invisible beauty is now demonstrated.

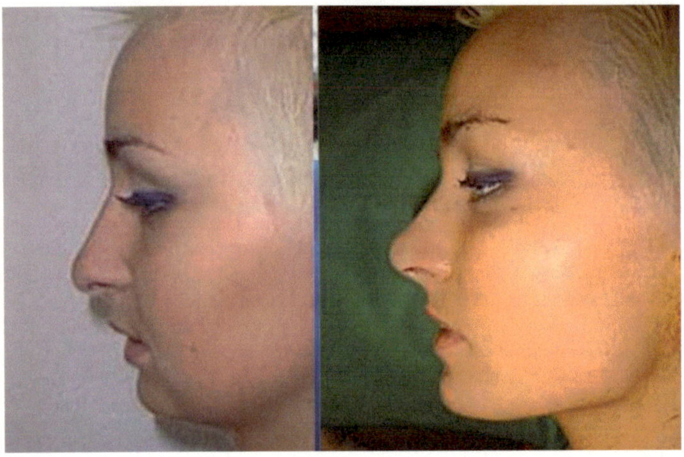

A. B.

Figure 9. Immediate result (Braunol disinfection is still not totally cleaned) after nasal tip rotation by T-excision and chin enhancement by Serdev Suture® in a case of a long nose, small chin (retrognatia), and improper ratio in the lower part of the face (between upper lip and chin); **A.** Before. The upper face is nice, but the nose is long, the chin is small and disproportional. Straight line of the noble profile is missing. Due to short mandible and reduced skeleton support, surrounding and submandibular tissue is hanging; **B.** After. Immediate result after T-excision for nasal tip rotation, columella sliding for tip projection and chin augmentation collecting her own tissue using Serdev Suture® volumizing method. Correct volumes are visible – nasal tip on the line of the cheekbone prominence. The result includes: proper

http://dx.doi.org/10.5772/62061

aesthetic proportions of the face (three equal parts of the face); tip is correctly rotated; and the nose is proportional. The tip is projected to fit to the proper 30^0 dorsoprofile angle; the chin is augmented using her own collected tissue, without foreign materials; jaw line and submandibular line are stretched; lower face proportions are corrected: lip to chin ratio (incl. lower lip) is 1:2; straight noble profile is present. The immediate result presents the beauty of the face.

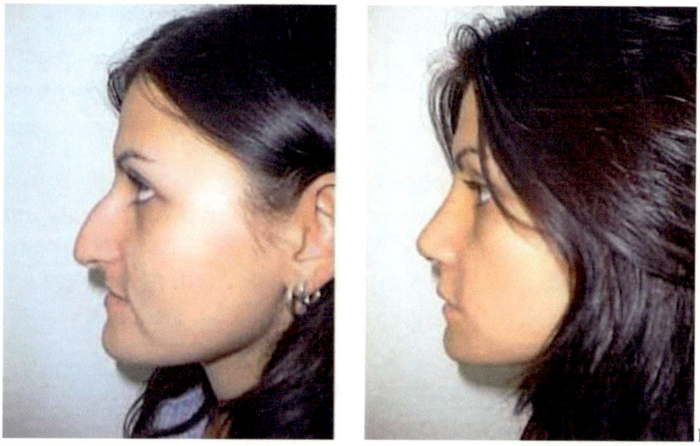

A. B.

Figure 10. A. Before. Aquiline long nose, short upper lip, and prognatic jaw. **B.** One year after T-excision for nasal tip rotation, humpectomy, digital fracture instead of lateral osteotomy, caudal septum and nasal spine resection for upper lip elongation, upper lip volumizing by Serdev Suture®. Changes include: proper angles of the nose; it occupies 1/3 of the face, correct aesthetic proportions of the face (three equal parts); the upper lip is elongated and brought forward (thus, the prognatic jaw is included in the correct proportions); proportions of the lower face are in a good ratio; a straight noble profile is present. The result is beautification of the face.

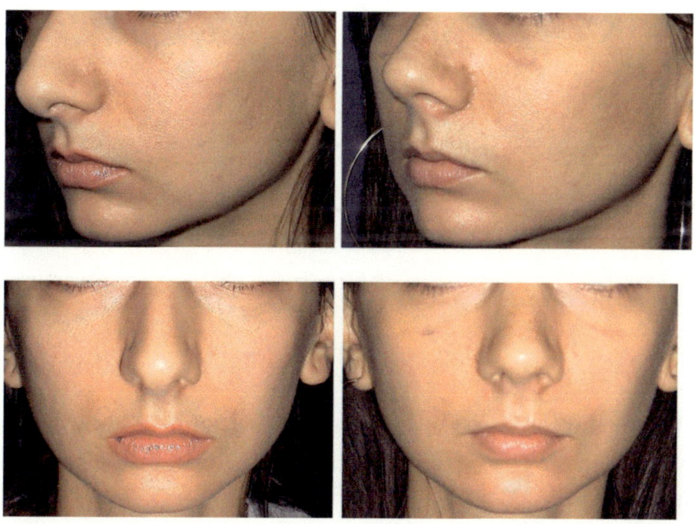

Figure 11. A disproportionally long nose is shortened by tip rotation via T-excision to obtain 3 equal parts of the face with correct angles of the nose.

7. Conclusion

Beautification is a work of art. Rhinoplasty, including shortening of a long nose, aims at obtaining exact aesthetic proportions, volumes, and angles of the face. The nose cannot be separated aesthetically. T-excision en bloc, including cephalic strip and elongated caudal septum resection can rotate the nasal tip to obtain correct proportions of the face. The procedure takes a very short time, even shorter than a medical injection rhinoplasty. It is atraumatic, nearly bloodless, does not require plaster fixation, tampons, and downtime. The results are permanent.

Patients return to work and social life almost immediately. There is no bruising. Edema is not visible for observers. Swelling can minimally change the tip position only in the first 5–7 days. After that it becomes natural and in the right position. T-excision is the shortest rhinoplasty procedure to correct long noses and dropping columella, with the most stable and permanent results, due to very small or lack of trauma to the greater alar cartilages and surrounding tissue.

7.1. In cases of over-rotation or short upper lip

If the upper lip is shortened by a too long septum or shortening of the whole pyramid of the nose is necessary, the prominent posterior septal angle can be excised, together with the prominence of the anterior nasal spine. This maneuver deepens the nasolabial angle. It elongates the upper lip and can also correct an over-rotated nasal tip (see Chapter 2)

Author details

Nikolay P. Serdev*

Address all correspondence to: serdev@gmail.com

New Bulgarian University, Sofia, Medical Centre "Aesthetic Surgery and Aesthetic Medicine," Sofia, Bulgaria

References

[1] Serdev NP. Principles of Face Beautification. Ier Congreso International De Medicina y Cirugia Cosmetica, The South American Academy of Cosmetic Surgery, Buenos Aires – Argentina, Oct. 31–Nov. 1, 1999

[2] Serdev NP. Sliding of the Columella by the Serdev Technique. Live Surgery Workshop, The International Academy of Aesthetic Surgery and Aesthetic Medicine, Krulig Clinic, Caracas, Venezuela, Nov. 1999

[3] Serdev NP. Principles of Face Beautification. Third World Congress of the International Society of Aesthetic Surgery, Tokyo April 8-10, 2000

[4] Serdev NP. Rhinoplasty for Beautification. Asia Pacific Craniofacial Association. Third Conference, Shanghai, P.R. China, Oct. 30–Nov. 1, 2000

[5] Serdev NP. Beautification rhinoplasty. *Int J Cosm Surg* 2001; 1(3): 257-311

[6] Serdev NP. Aesthetic surgery methods for face beautification. *Int J Cosm Surg* 2001; 1(3): 188-256

[7] Serdev NP. Serdev techniques in beautification rhinoplasty: T-zone excision, columella sliding, Serdev sutures. *Int J Cosm Surg* 2008; 8(1):388-469

[8] Serdev NP. Nasal tip refinement, rotation, projection, alar base narrowing In: Serdev NP, Ed. *Serdev Sutures® Face and Body Lifts and/or Volumising*. Marllor editions, Italy, 2013: 75-81

[9] Serdev NP. Serdev Sutures® in middle face 4. Beautification rhinoplasty – tip rotation and refinement, alar base narrowing. In: Serdev NP, Ed. *Miniinvasive Face and Body Lifts – Closed Suture Lifts or Barded Thread Lifts*. Intech, Rijeka, 2013. Available from http://www.intechopen.com/books/miniinvasive-face-and-body-lifts-closed-suture-lifts-or-barbed-thread-lifts/serdev-sutures-in-middle-face.

[10] Daniel RK. Tip. In: *Rhinoplasty: An Atlas of Surgical Techniques*. New York, Springer-Verlag New York Inc; 2002; pp. 59-139

Excision of Prominent Posterior Septal Angle and Nasal Spine for Downward Tip Rotation, in Short Upper Lip, or Over-Rotated Tip

Nikolay P. Serdev

Additional information is available at the end of the chapter

http://dx.doi.org/10.5772/62062

Abstract

The author uses resection of the posterior septal angle and nasal spine for downward tip rotation in cases of obtuse nasolabial angle and a short upper lip [1-8]. It could be an independent procedure or part of T-excision, or other type of primary or secondary rhinoplasty. This excision is easy to perform, prolonging the retrocolumellar incision downward. A 2–3 mm excision of the length of the caudal septum in the part of the posterior septal angle (including the spina nasalis anterior) may be enough to shorten the length of the nasal pyramid at its base and adapt the long pyramid to the aesthetic middle-third of the face. This is helpful especially in women with delicate faces and unproportional noses. This procedure is mini-invasive, nearly bloodless, does not require tampons or bandages. There is almost no downtime.

Keywords: Rhinoplasty, excision, posterior septal angle, nasal spine, mini-invasive technique, long nose, elongated septum, over-rotated tip, short upper lip, primary or secondary, retrocolumellar incision, no bandages, no downtime

1. Introduction

If the upper lip is shortened by a too long septum, or if shortening of the longer nasal pyramid is necessary, the prominent posterior septal angle can be excised, together with the anterior nasal spine [4]. This maneuver deepens the nasolabial angle and can be used also in cases of over-rotated tip (obtuse tip).

2. Anatomy

The length of the nasal pyramid should occupy the middle-third of the face. Longer pyramid should be shortened, if unproportional to the face. This could happen when reducing the prominent posterior septal angle and the prominence of the anterior nasal spine.

In long and aquiline noses the facial proportions are imbalanced. Often, except the elongation of the caudal septum, the nasal pyramid (including the posterior septal angle) and nasal spine can also be elongated with shortening of the upper lip. In these cases cephalic strip excision alone does not suffice to shorten the elongated nasal pyramid.

Vice versa, in Asian and Afro-American noses, as well as in some secondary iatrogenic cases, the tip can be over-rotated with an obtuse nasolabial angle, which could be a good indication for excision of the prominent posterior septal angle and anterior nasal spine.

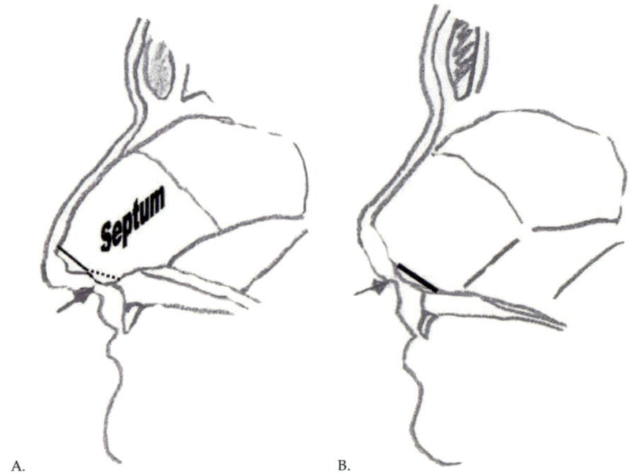

Figure 1. A: Long aquiline nose, Short upper lip, elongated septal cartilage, and nasal pyramid. Author's T-excision, or cephalic strip excision and caudal septal shortening could help in this case, together with posterior septal angle and nasal spine resection (marked) to elongate the upper lip. **B.** Ethnic (Asian or Afro-American) or iatrogenic obtuse nasolabial angle with over-rotated tip. Precise excision of the posterior septal angle and nasal spine (marked) can help to correct the nasolabial and tip angle.

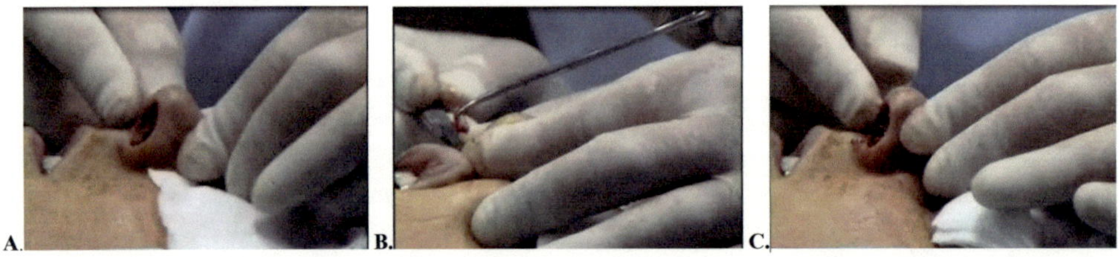

Figure 2. A: Prominent posterior septal angle and nasal spine. **B.** 2-3 mm excision of the posterior septal angle incl. nasal spine. **C.** Correct position of the posterior septal angle.

3. Indications

Ethnic aquiline long noses with elongated nasal pyramid as well as ethnic (Asian or Afro-American) or iatrogenic over-rotated tip with obtuse nasolabial angle.

4. Surgical technique

It is an outpatient technique under local anesthesia. It could be performed as an independent procedure in cases of iatrogenic or ethnic over-rotated tips as well as in case of long or aquiline noses.

In all cases, a retrocolumellar incision is performed, which will be prolonged downward to excise about 2 mm, rarely 3 mm, of the posterior septal angle together with the anterior nasal spine.

The author fixes the columella to the septum with transmucosal mattress sutures, which remain for 2–3 weeks. No bandages or tampons are necessary for this separate procedure. It is mini-invasive, atraumatic, and bloodless.

5. Clinical cases

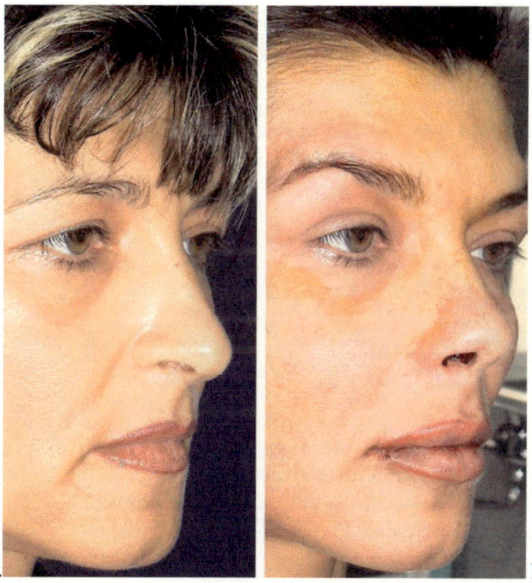

Figure 3. A. Before. Long nose and proportionally shortened upper lip. **B.** Immediately after T-excision for tip rotation to obtain correct aesthetic proportions of the face, combined with a 2 mm excision of the prominent posterior septal angle and nasal spine (for elongation of the upper lip and achieving a correct proportion of the lower face). Simultaneous brow lift and lip augmentation. The picture is taken in the operation room. The face is still not cleaned from the Braunol disinfection.

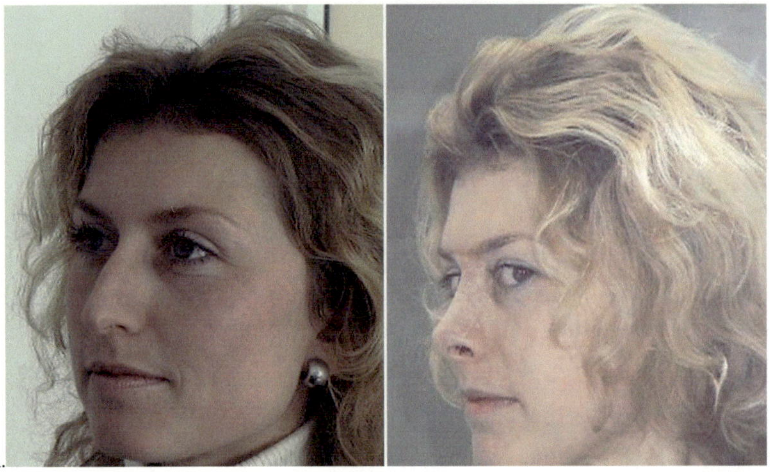

A. B.

Figure 4. A. Before. Ethnic long and aquiline nose, disrupting the correct facial proportions. Short upper lip, with incorrect 3:1 proportion of the lower face. **B.** After. Rhinoplasty, including humpectomy, digital fracture vs. lateral osteotomy, T-excision for tip rotation and 3 mm excision of the prominent posterior septal angle and nasal spine. The result is correct aesthetic proportions of the face and lower third of the face. The photo is taken in the operation theater, immediately after ambulatory closed rhinoplasty – atraumatic, mini-invasive, bloodless. The result is beautification.

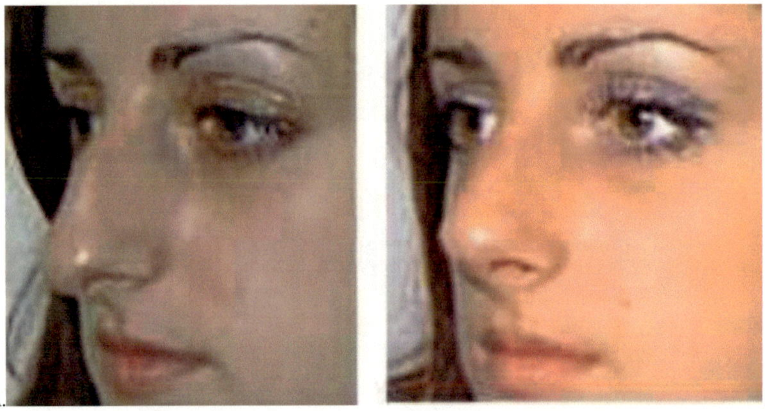

A. B.

Figure 5. A. Before. Ethnic long and aquiline nose disrupting the correct facial proportions. No self-confidence, uncertain appearance. Short upper lip. **B.** After. Rhinoplasty, including humpectomy, digital fracture vs. lateral osteotomy, T-excision for tip rotation and 3 mm excision of the prominent posterior septal angle and nasal spine to improve the lower third of the face. The result is beautification and improved self-confidence.

6. Conclusion

Excision of caudal septum in long noses, combined with excision of prominent posterior septal angle and nasal spine, is a very effective technique. It is of great help in cases of longer caudal

http://dx.doi.org/10.5772/62062

septum and nasal pyramid with a short upper lip, as well as in cases of over-rotated noses. The procedure helps to adapt the face to correct aesthetic proportions, which is the main goal in beautification. The technique itself is time-saving, atraumatic, and also very well tolerated by patients, with no downtime and immediate return to work and social life.

Author details

Nikolay P. Serdev*

Address all correspondence to: serdev@gmail.com

New Bulgarian University, Sofia, Medical Centre "Aesthetic Surgery and Aesthetic Medicine," Sofia, Bulgaria

References

[1] Serdev NP. Sliding of the columella by the Serdev Technique, Live Surgery Workshop, The International Academy of Aesthetic Surgery and Aesthetic Medicine, Krulig Clinic, Caracas, Venezuela, Nov. 1999

[2] Serdev NP. Principles of Face Beautification, Third World Congress of the International Society of Aesthetic Surgery, Tokyo, April 8-10, 2000

[3] Serdev NP. Rhinoplasty for Beautification. Asia Pacific Craniofacial Association. Third Conference, Shanghai, P.R. China, Oct. 30–Nov. 1, 2000

[4] Serdev NP. Beautification rhinoplasty. *Int J Cosm Surg* 2006; 6(1): 1-53

[5] Serdev NP. Serdev techniques in beautification rhinoplasty: T-zone excision, columella sliding, Serdev sutures. *Int J Cosm Surg* 2008; 8(1):388-469

[6] Serdev NP. Nasal tip refinement, rotation, projection, alar base narrowing In: Serdev NP, Ed. *Serdev Sutures® Face and Body Lifts and/or Volumising*. Marllor editions, Italy, 2013: 75-81

[7] Serdev NP. Serdev Sutures® in middle face 4. Beautification rhinoplasty – tip rotation and refinement, alar base narrowing. In: Serdev NP, Ed. *Miniinvasive Face and Body Lifts – Closed Suture Lifts or Barded Thread Lifts*. Intech, Rijeka, 2013. Available from http://www.intechopen.com/books/miniinvasive-face-and-body-lifts-closed-suture-lifts-or-barbed-thread-lifts/serdev-sutures-in-middle-face.

[8] Serdev NP. Course: Beautification rhinoplasty, t-zone excision, columella sliding, suture methods, Updates in IV sedation and analgesia. 2005; Feb. 23. Available from: http://ijcs.org/courses/2005/90/index.php

Chapter 3

Columella Sliding for Nasal Tip Projection Using Septocolumellar Transmucosal Mattress Sutures

Nikolay P. Serdev

Additional information is available at the end of the chapter

http://dx.doi.org/10.5772/62063

Abstract

In author's hands, columella sliding is a surgical technique to correct unaesthetic/unwanted depression or projection of the nasal tip. The tip can be increased or decreased by a simple mini-invasive technique during primary or secondary rhinoplasty as well as by a separate procedure. Main aim of the technique is to obtain the aesthetic 30° angle between dorsum and profile line and correct volume of the nasal tip at the line of the beauty triangle. It is possible to change the projection of the nasal tip using a retrocolumellar incision, to slide columella against septum upward or downward and fix the new position with 2–3 transmucosal columella-septal sutures. The stitches will be removed after 2–3 weeks, which is enough for columella to heal stable initially to septum. Columella sliding is an important technique to obtain a dorsoprofile angle of 30°, which is an aesthetic rule. The technique is atraumatic, mini-invasive, nearly bloodless. The procedure is very well tolerated by patients: there is no need of casts, tampons, and patients return to social life almost immediately.

Keywords: Rhinoplasty, columella sliding, retrocolumellar incision, columella-septal incision, mattress transmucosal suture, columella sliding upward, columella sliding downward, no downtime, atraumatic

1. Introduction

1.1. Surgical procedure

Nasal tip projection determines how far out from the face the tip protrudes. The author accepts that the correct position of the nasal tip is in close relation to the 30^0 dorsoprofile or dorsoalar angle [1-5], where the alar line refers to a vertical line drawn through the point where the alar base attaches to the cheek and establishes the straight profile line. A 30^0 dorsoalar angle is accepted as aesthetic.

When a retrocolumellar incision is present, 2–3 mattress transmucosal sutures are passed from columella caudal surface to a higher point of caudal septum to give projection to the nasal tip. (Figure 1). Vice versa, the columella is sutured to lower points of the septum to lower the projection of the tip in selected cases. The suture is used as well in cases of hanging columella after artistic excision of retrocolumellar mucosa and eventually part of caudally projected septum. The sutures are removed after 2 weeks. This time is observed to be enough to form a stable fibrosis and give a permanent result. Patients have to prevent the nasal tip from trauma. The depressor septi nasi muscle is responsible for smiling deformity. Excision of the depressor nasi muscle or botox injections could help additionally in this regard. Patients are asked to reduce wide opening of the mouth and too much laughing, in order to prevent from depressing the tip during the early post-op and healing period.

The author has experienced no complication with any of the above-described transcutaneous and transmucosal sutures in more than a thousand operated cases. Sutures can be placed at any time as ambulatory procedures with no downtime.

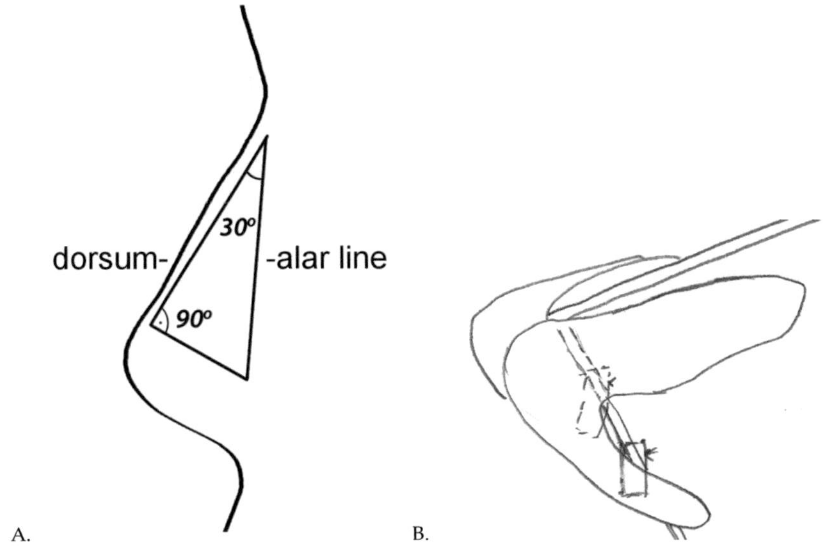

Figure 1. A. The position of the nasal tip implements the proper formation of the 30° dorsoalar angle, which is responsible for how far from the face the tip is positioned. **B.** When a retrocolumellar incision is present, 2–3 mattress transmucosal sutures are passed from columella caudal surface to a higher point of caudal septum to give projection to the tip. Vice versa, the columella is sutured to lower points of the septum to lower the projection of the tip in selected cases. The suture is used as well in cases of hanging columella after artistic excision of retrocolumellar mucosa and eventually part of caudally projected septum.

2. Clinical cases

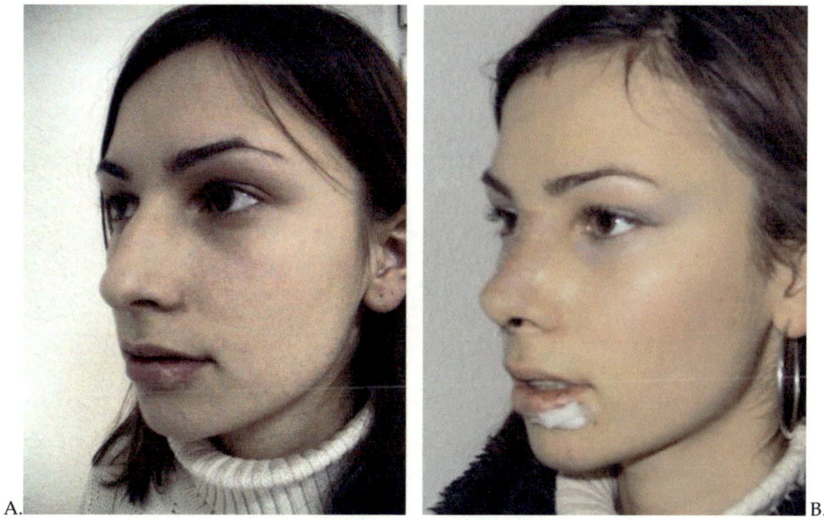

Figure 2. A. Before. Aquiline long nose. No aesthetic proportions are present. B. After. Day 1 after T-excision for nasal tip rotation, humpectomy, digital fracture, and columella sliding for exact tip projection; simultaneous chin augmentation by Serdev Suture® and lower lip scar excision. Atraumatic surgery, no plaster, no tampons. The skin color tape will be removed on day 3. There is no bruising due to atraumatic technique. On day 1, patients visit the clinic to clean the nose, remove the crust. On the question why she has used make up, she answered that she feels beautiful.

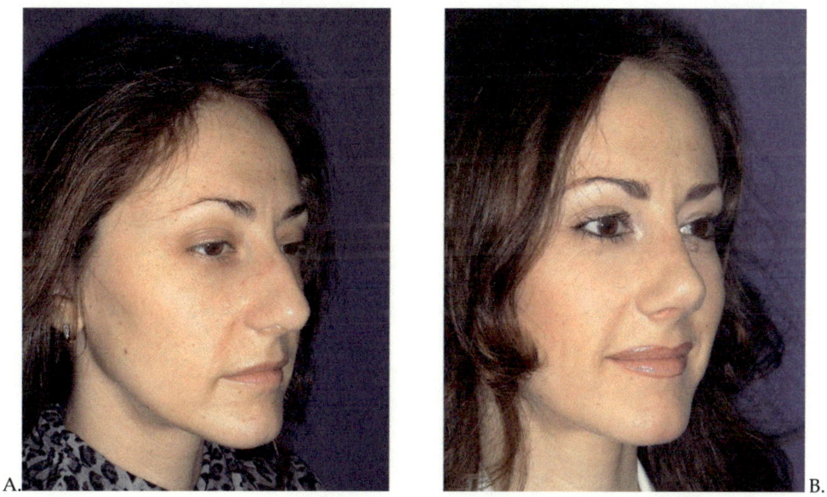

Figure 3. A. Before. Aquiline long nose. No aesthetic proportions are present. B. Day 4 after T-excision for nasal tip rotation, humpectomy, digital fracture, and columella sliding for exact tip projection. Better self-confidence, still some nearly invisible edema, no bruising. Beautification without additional surgeries due to correct proportions, volumes, and angles.

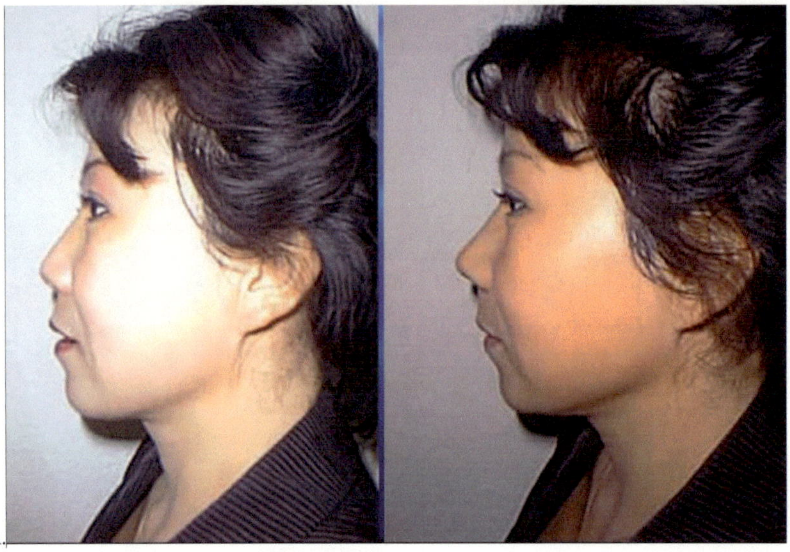

A. B.

Figure 4. A. Before. Asian patient with a typical, very acute dorsoprofile angle, and low position of the nasal tip. **B.** After columella sliding for tip projection as a separate procedure. A correct 30^0 dorsoprofile angle is obtained, which changes positively the flat appearance of the Asian face.

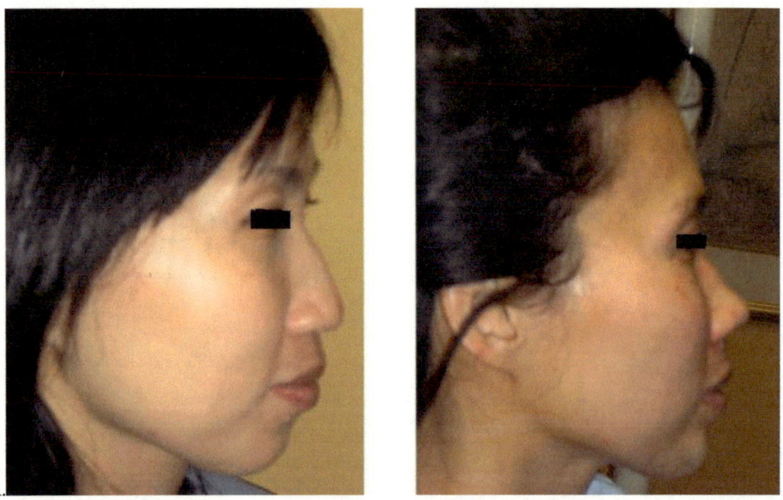

A. B.

Figure 5. A. Asian patient with an aquiline long nose and retrograde chin. **B.** Immediately after T-excision for nasal tip rotation, columella sliding for tip projection, and chin enhancement with Serdev Suture® for straight profile. Correct proportions, volumes, and angles lead to beautification.

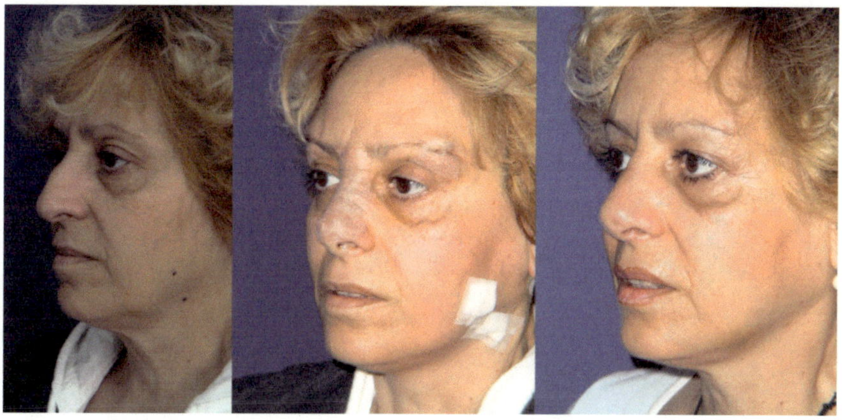

Figure 6. A. Before. Aging face and aquiline long nose. No aesthetic proportions are present. **B.** Immediatelly after Serdev Suture® temporal, medial, and lower face and neck lifts, and rhinoplasty: T-excision for nasal tip rotation, humpectomy, digital fracture, and columella sliding for tip projection. **C.** After 18 months. Correct proportions and dorsoprofile angle. Rejuvenation and beautification are present.

A.

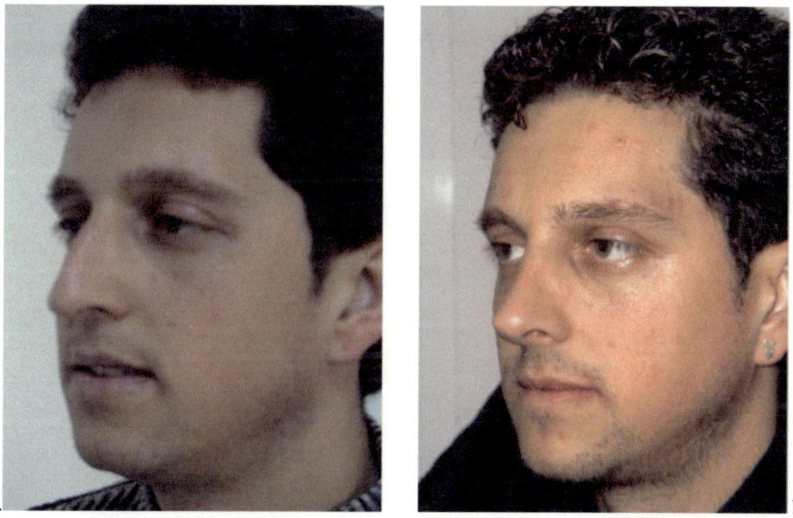

B.

Figure 7. A. Before. Incorrect proportions, Aquiline long nose, low eyebrows, retrograde chin. **B.** After rhinoplasty including T-excision, humpectomy, digital fracture and columella sliding for correct proportion and angles, along with simultaneous brow lift and chin enhancement using Serdev Suture® techniques. Beautification as a result of correct proportions, volumes, and angles.

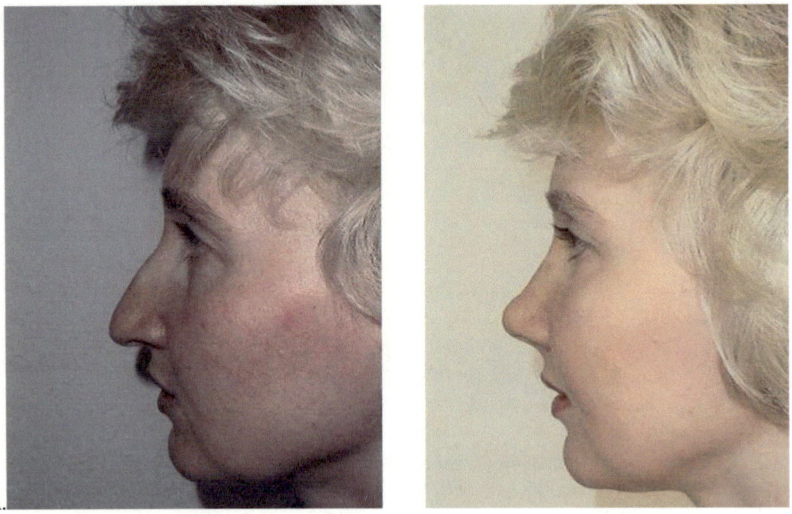

A. B.

Figure 8. A. Before. Incorrect proportions, aquiline long nose. **B.** After rhinoplasty, including T-excision, humpectomy, digital fracture and columella sliding for correct proportion and angles. Beautification as a result of correct proportions, volumes, and angles.

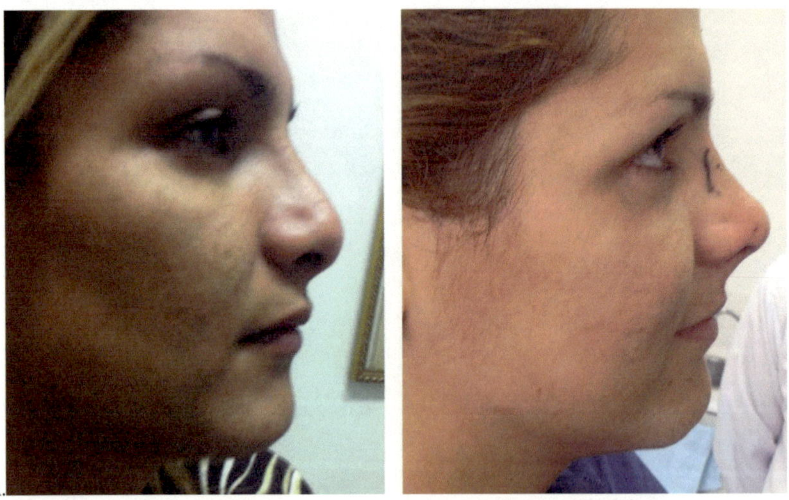

A. B.

Figure 9. A. Before. Secondary case with short columella and incorrect acute dorsoprofile angle. **B.** After columella sliding for correct nasal tip projection and dorsoprofile angle of 30^0.

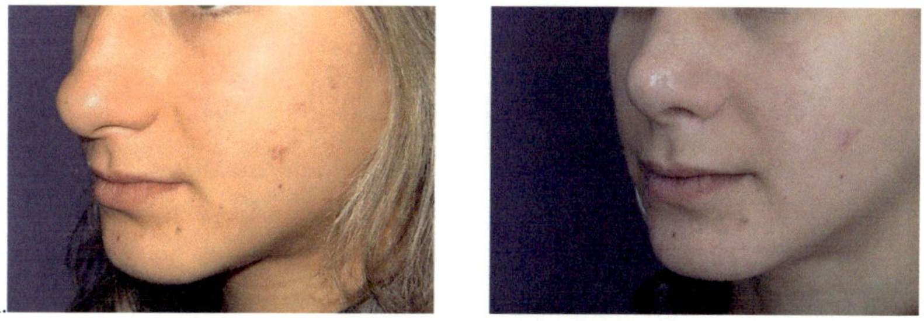

Figure 10. A. Before. Incorrect proportions, long nose with a bulbous tip and columella hanging.. **B.** After rhinoplasty, including T-excision, humpectomy, digital fracture, and columella sliding downward for correct reduction of the nasal tip projection.

3. Conclusion

Columella sliding is a very useful mini-invasive technique to control position of the nasal tip as an independent procedure or as a part of primary or secondary rhinoplasties. It is simple, atraumatic, and very well accepted by patients. There are no known complications and the columella is fixed and heals in the new position in 2–3 weeks. There is no bruising, no need of tapes, tampons, or casts. Downtime is minimal and patients can return to social life almost immediately.

Author details

Nikolay P. Serdev*

Address all correspondence to: serdev@gmail.com

New Bulgarian University, Sofia, Medical Centre "Aesthetic Surgery and Aesthetic Medicine," Sofia, Bulgaria

References

[1] Serdev NP. Sliding of the Columella by the Serdev Technique. Live Surgery Workshop, The International Academy of Aesthetic Surgery and Aesthetic Medicine, Krulig Clinic, Caracas, Venezuela, Nov. 1999

[2] Serdev NP. Principles of Face Beautification. Third World Congress of the International Society of Aesthetic Surgery, Tokyo April 8-10, 2000

[3] Serdev NP. Rhinoplasty for Beautification. Asia Pacific Craniofacial Association. Third Conference, Shanghai, P.R. China, Oct. 30–Nov. 1, 2000

[4] Serdev NP. Beautification rhinoplasty. *Int J Cosm Surg* 2001; 1(3): 257-311

[5] Serdev NP. Aesthetic surgery methods for face beautification. *Int J Cosm Surg* 2001; 1(3): 188-256

[6] Serdev NP. Serdev techniques in beautification rhinoplasty: T-zone excision, columella sliding, Serdev sutures. *Int J Cosm Surg* 2008; 8(1):388-469

[7] Serdev NP. Nasal tip refinement, rotation, projection, alar base narrowing In: Serdev NP, Ed. *Serdev Sutures® Face and Body Lifts and/or Volumising*. Marllor editions, Italy, 2013: 75-81

[8] Serdev NP. Serdev Sutures® in middle face 4. Beautification rhinoplasty – tip rotation and refinement, alar base narrowing. In: Serdev NP, Ed. *Miniinvasive Face and Body Lifts – Closed Suture Lifts or Barded Thread Lifts*. Intech, Rijeka, 2013. Available from http://www.intechopen.com/books/miniinvasive-face-and-body-lifts-closed-suture-lifts-or-barbed-thread-lifts/serdev-sutures-in-middle-face.

[9] Serdev NP. Course: Beautification rhinoplasty, t-zone excision, columella sliding, suture methods, updates in IV sedation and analgesia 2005; 23. 02. Available from: http://ijcs.org/courses/2005/90/index.php

Chapter 4

Digital Fracture Versus Lateral Osteotomy

Nikolay P. Serdev

Additional information is available at the end of the chapter

http://dx.doi.org/10.5772/62064

Abstract

The purpose of digital fracture versus lateral osteotomies is to narrow the bony base of the nose after the dorsal correction, by closing the open dorsal roof, avoiding the lateral "rocker" or steplike deformities. The author presents the digital fracture technique, which is simple, safer, closes the open dorsal roof after medial osteotomy much better, and does not provoke bleeding and bruising. It is atraumatic and saves time during the operation and recovery.

Keywords: Rhinoplasty, digital fracture, infracture versus lateral osteotomy, dorsal roof closure, mini- invasive, atraumatic, no bleeding, small bruising, no complications

1. Introduction

Lateral osteotomy, internal or external, or in different levels, has some negatives that can lead to single or multiple reoperations. Its main complications are: unnatural contour of nasal bones; visible and palpable bony step, collapse of the upper lateral cartilages, along with infection, bleeding, massive edema, anosmia, lacrimal duct injury, intracranial injuries, disfigured appearance, narrow airway, and nasal obstruction. It is very difficult to reverse a lateral osteotomy and revision may end up with more of a flat top or square top nose, known as an open roof deformity [1, 2].

Choosing a method for closure of the open dorsal roof after medial osteotomy must be balanced with the other features and characteristics of the nose. In this regard, "digital fracture" has many advantages over lateral osteotomy – it is much more precise in closing the dorsal roof, without danger of bleeding, step formation, collapse of the upper lateral cartilages, and nasal obstruction. It is performed easily in any type of nose. The author has not observed any complications connected to this technique [3, 4].

2. Surgical technique

The author applies the digital fracture technique after medial osteotomy and hump removal, in primary as well as in secondary cases. It is performed by applying lateral pressure on the nasal bone in its dorsocaudal end, using the thumb. The other hand fixes the head with opposite pressure (Figure 1). There is a very small percentage of difficult digital fractures, mostly in men with thick nasal bones. A skin-colored tape is used for 3 days to reduce the swelling – the glue of the tape is hypertensive and partially absorbs the edema (Figure 2).

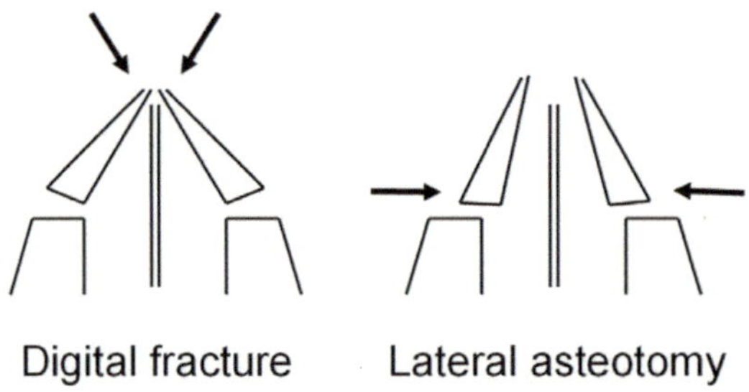

Figure 1. Digital fracture better adapts the nasal bones to close the dorsum and prevents step form deformity, which can often be seen in cases with lateral osteotomies.

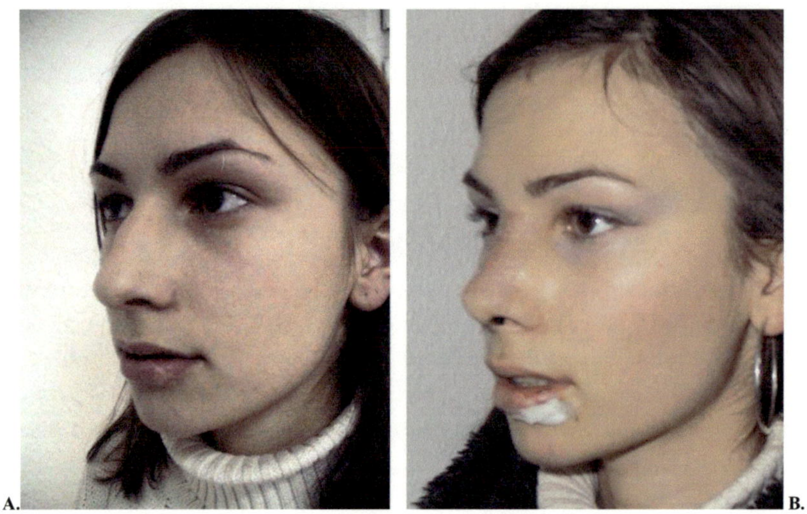

Figure 2. A. Before. Aquiline long nose. No aesthetic proportions are present. **B.** After. Day 1 after T-excision for nasal tip rotation, humpectomy, digital fracture, and columella sliding for exact tip projection; simultaneous chin augmentation by Serdev Suture® and lower lip scar excision. Atraumatic surgery, no plaster, no tampons. Aesthetic proportions, angles, and volumes give aesthetic beautification The skin-colored tape will be removed on day 3. On day 1, as apparent, there is no bruising due to the atraumatic nature of the technique. On the first day, patients visit the clinic to have their nose cleaned and the crust removed. On questioning why she has used make up, she answered that she feels beautiful.

The technique has been used in all cases of author's rhinoplasties with humpectomy, under local anesthesia, since 1994. It gives a very natural result in all primary cases, as well as in secondary cases. It saves time, there is almost no bleeding and trauma is minimal Thus, downtime is shortened.

3. Clinical cases

In all of author's chapters, results after humpectomy show the result of digital fracture as well.

Due to the lack of trauma, there is no post-op bruising in 30% of the cases with medial osteotomy and digital fracture.

Bruising is observed in nearly 70% of the cases. It is mostly linear along the tear through and disappears in a week (Figure 3).

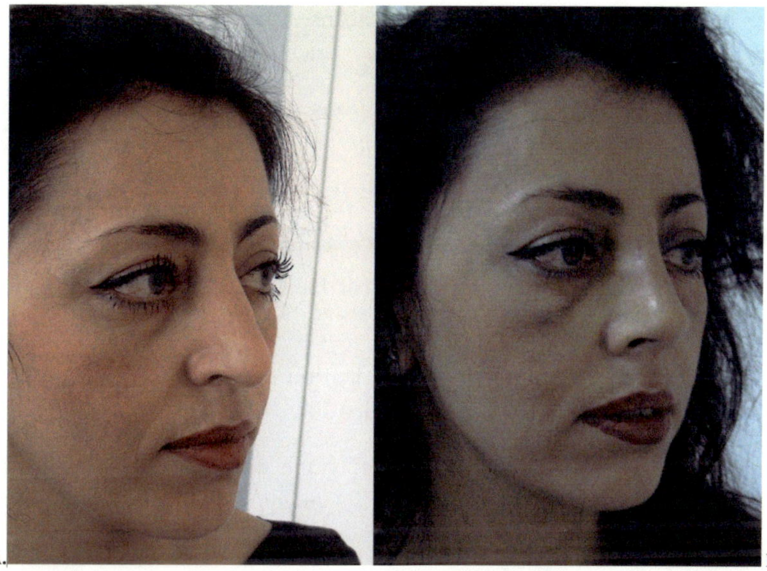

A. B.

Figure 3. A. Before. A patient with a so-called Greek long nose. Small hump is present with no marked nasion concavity. **B**. Third day after humpectomy and digital fracture of the nasal bones, T-excision and columella sliding. The nasion is marked, the dorsum is slightly concave. Beautification is visible, due to correct aesthetic proportions, nasal angles, and tip volume. On the third day post op, the tape is removed, edema and bruising are minimal.

4. Conclusions

Digital fracture is superior to lateral osteotomy. It is a very simple technique, atraumatic, takes only some minutes to perform, prevents from bleeding and shortens downtime. It prevents surgeons and patients from all possible lateral osteotomy complications and has no known complications itself.

Author details

Nikolay P. Serdev*

Address all correspondence to: serdev@gmail.com

New Bulgarian University, Sofia, Medical Centre "Aesthetic Surgery and Aesthetic Medicine," Sofia, Bulgaria

References

[1] Rolling KD. Primary rhinoplasty. Osteotomies. In: Rolling KD, Ed. *Rhinoplasty: An Atlas of Surgical Technique*. Springer, New York, 1999: 304.

[2] Trenité GJ. Surgery of the osseocartilaginous vault. Osteotomies. In: Trenité GJ, Ed. *Rhinoplasty: A Practical Guide to Functional and Aesthetic Surgery of the Nose*. Kugler publications, The Hague, 2005: 102.

[3] Serdev NP. Beautification rhinoplasty. *Int J Cosm Surg* 2001; 1(3): 257-311

[4] Serdev NP. Aesthetic surgery methods for face beautification. *Int J Cosm Surg* 2001; 1(3): 188-256

[5] Serdev NP. Serdev techniques in beautification rhinoplasty: T-zone excision, columella sliding, Serdev sutures. *Int J Cosm Surg* 2008; 8(1):388-469

[6] Serdev NP. Nasal tip refinement, rotation, projection, alar base narrowing In: Serdev NP, Ed. *Serdev Sutures® Face and Body Lifts and/or Volumising*. Marllor editions, Italy, 2013: 75-81

[7] Serdev NP. Serdev Sutures® in middle face 4. Beautification rhinoplasty – tip rotation and refinement, alar base narrowing. In: Serdev NP, Ed. *Miniinvasive Face and Body Lifts – Closed Suture Lifts or Barded Thread Lifts*. Intech, Rijeka, 2013. Available from http://www.intechopen.com/books/miniinvasive-face-and-body-lifts-closed-suture-lifts-or-barbed-thread-lifts/serdev-sutures-in-middle-face.

[8] Serdev NP. Secondary rhinoplasty - Tip rotation by Serdev suture after hump removal (video) YouTube 2011; 12.04. Available from http://www.youtube.com/watch?v=nRh8NDSgDck

[9] Serdev NP. Beautification rhinoplasty in a long nose t excision columella sliding 26.10.2013 r. http://www.youtube.com/watch?v=v1wMYoOayKc

Chapter 5

Debridement of Lower Lateral Cartilages in Cleft Lip–Nose Cases along with Management of Skin and Fibrotic Traction

Nikolay P. Serdev

Additional information is available at the end of the chapter

http://dx.doi.org/10.5772/62075

Abstract

Rhinoplasties in case of cleft lip–nose and palate are difficult and may include: primary repair of nasal deformities at the time of cleft lip repair; secondary staged repair of cleft lip–nasal deformities; separation of the quadrangular cartilage of the septum from the maxillary crest and securing it to the midline; removal of deviated portions, strut grafts, transplants to project the radix and dorsum, cartilage grafts, multidisciplinary care, etc. Results can vary widely, from excellent in primary corrections to very poor in late surgery cases. In some secondary rhinoplasties, based on skin and fibrotic tractions and deviations, the author offers a more simple method of debridement of the normally formed cartilages. It includes closed approach T-excision with releasing the alar cartilages from their attachments, columella sliding and sutures for stabilization of the columella, nasal tip refinement, dorsal augmentation, and overall symmetry. Such approach could be sufficient in selected cases. In other cases, additional steps may be necessary.

Keywords: Rhinoplasty, cleft lip and nose, debridement, T-excision, transcutaneous Serdev Sutures®, symmetrization, parallel medial crura suture, columella sliding for tip projection

1. Introduction

The goal of surgical treatment of cleft nasal deformity is not only rhinoplasty but includes normal speech, aesthetic facial appearance, normal occlusion, unobstructed nasal passages, and absence of psychological pathology. Surgical correction of nasal deformities removes the abnormal appearance and improves the opportunities for normal social integration.

2. Secondary rhinoplasty

Despite the move toward primary correction of cleft nasal deformities, secondary rhinoplasty procedures are often necessary. It is advisable that the patient has reached bony maturity. Maxillary deficiencies have to be treated appropriately prior to surgery.

Open approach is often used, because it provides exposure. Autologous cartilage grafts are often used to provide structural support and to restore contours and grafts – to project and support.

3. Surgical technique

Having in mind that deformations depend mostly on skin/fibrotic traction, the author uses the closed rhinoplasty approach. Its main goals, by steps, are:

1. Using retrocolumellar incision and eventually T-excision technique to correct hanging columella or elongated (mostly deviated) caudal septum.

2. To release the lower lateral cartilages from the skin/fibrotic lateral attachments and reposition them. Usually, alar cartilages show minimal deformations.

3. To redefine the dome and tip defining points, using transcutaneous Serdev Sutures® (described in the next chapter): a. for tip refinement and symmetrization of the tip and tip defining points of projection; b. transmucosal domal and columellar sutures for refinement of the nasal tip and stabilization of the columella. In cases of equal projection of both sides of the tip, the needle should penetrate horizontally. The trick to get symmetry in unequal projection of both sides is to place the needle and suture parallel to the asymmetric tip (Figure 1).

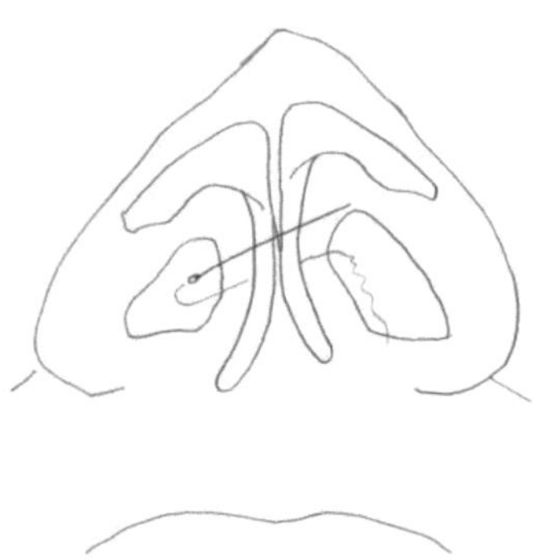

Figure 1. Transmucosal sutures have to be parallel to the symmetry or asymmetry of the tip defining points; 2–3 sutures can equalize the dome projection on both sides.

4. To project the nasal tip. Instead of a columellar strut graft, the author uses columella sliding for nasal tip projection. Note that columella sliding cannot be used in most Asian, Afro-American, and some Latino-American patients, where the columella is typically soft and unstable and is the main reason for the low projection in these ethnic groups. Caucasian septum and columella are very stable and in most cases do not need additional support.

Repositioning of the lower lateral cartilage and some of the described mini-invasive techniques can be sufficient to restore the columella, refine the nasal tip, get tip projection, and achieve overall symmetry (Figure 2).

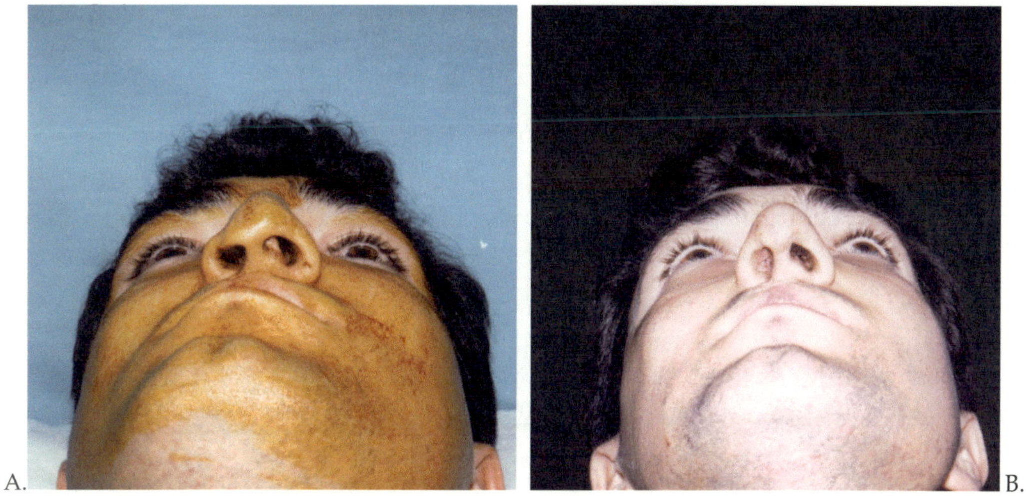

Figure 2. A. Before. The lower lateral cartilages in cleft lip and nose cases are exposed to skin/fibrotic pressure and/or traction. The chin is deviated to the right. **B**. After author's secondary rhinoplasty: retrocolumellar incision and T-excision technique to deal with hanging columella and elongated deviated caudal septum; debridement, release of lower lateral cartilages from the skin/fibrotic lateral attachments and their repositioning; transmucosal domal and columellar sutures to reposition the lower lateral cartilages and obtain symmetry at the domal tip **defining** points (as shown in Figure 1), for refinement of the tip and stabilization of the columella; redefining the dome and tip defining points using transcutaneous Serdev Sutures® (described in the next chapter) for tip refinement and **symmetrization** of the tip and tip defining points of projection; columella sliding for nasal tip projection. Additional Serdev Suture® technique is performed for transcutaneous chin soft tissue fixation to the left-side menton periosteum. The result is equalization and stabilization of the nose and overall facial symmetry.

More severe cases require additional procedures and local flaps for correction.

4. Conclusion

In selected cases, more atraumatic and mini-invasive techniques such as debridement and release of the lower lateral cartilages, author's suture techniques, and columella sliding can be enough to stabilize, equalize, and get overall symmetry of the nose and the whole face.

Author details

Nikolay P. Serdev*

Address all correspondence to: serdev@gmail.com

New Bulgarian University, Sofia, Medical Centre "Aesthetic Surgery and Aesthetic Medicine," Sofia, Bulgaria

References

[1] Serdev NP. Mentoplastia sin implantes. IX Journadas Mediteraneas de Confrontationes Terapeuticas an Medicina y Cirurgia Cosmetica, Sitges, Spain, May 2001. Available from: http://ijcs.org/7/23/135/index.php?pageFrom=1&pageTo=21

[2] Serdev NP. Principios basicos para el rejuvenecimiento facial. IX Journadas Mediteraneas de Confrontationes Terapeuticas an Medicina y Cirurgia Cosmetica, Sitges, Spain, May 2001. Available from: http://ijcs.org/7/23/128/index.php?pageFrom=1&pageTo=60

[3] Serdev NP. Suture Suspensions for Lifting or Volume Augmentation in Face and Body (English version), 2nd Annual Meeting of the National Bulgarian Society for Aesthetic Surgery and Aesthetic Medicine, Sofia, March 18, 1994, *Int J Aesth Cosm* 2001; 1(1):2561-2568

[4] Serdev NP. Principles of Face Beautification, Third World Congress of the International Society of Aesthetic Surgery, Tokyo April 8-10, 2000, 9W58

[5] Serdev NP. Serdev sutures for: Nasal tip refinement, nasal tip rotation, Nasal alar base narrowing. *Int J Cosm Surg* 2007; 7(1):328- 386

[6] Serdev NP. Serdev techniques in beautification rhinoplasty: T-zone excision, columella sliding, Serdev sutures. *Int J Cosm Surg* 2008; 8(1):388-469

[7] Serdev NP. Nasal tip refinement, rotation, projection, alar base narrowing In: Serdev NP, Ed. *Serdev Sutures® Face and Body Lifts and/or Volumising*. Marllor editions, Italy, 2013: 75-81

[8] Serdev NP. Serdev Sutures® in middle face 4. Beautification rhinoplasty – tip rotation and refinement, alar base narrowing. In: Serdev NP, Ed. *Miniinvasive Face and Body Lifts – Closed Suture Lifts or Barded Thread Lifts*. Intech, Rijeka, 2013. Available from http://www.intechopen.com/books/miniinvasive-face-and-body-lifts-closed-suture-lifts-or-barbed-thread-lifts/serdev-sutures-in-middle-face.

[9] Serdev NP. Live on TV Rhinoplasty, Brow Suture Lift, Chin Enhancement 10.01.2013 r. http://www.youtube.com/watch?v=H73PTB2xyKU

Transcutaneous and Transmucosal Serdev Sutures® for Nasal Tip Refinement, Alar Base Narrowing, and Other Corrections

Nikolay P. Serdev

Additional information is available at the end of the chapter

http://dx.doi.org/10.5772/62074

Abstract

The author describes his experience with the transcutaneous Serdev Suture® techniques in different aesthetic disproportions of the external nose and in secondary cases. Author's needles are specifically designed for these techniques. Rhinoplasty is part of the beautification process. The cosmetic surgeon should be guided by correct nose proportions, angles, and volumes. Proportional nose is one that fits in 1/3 of the face length. Proper volumes are: thin dorsum, thin tip, narrow alar base. The tip of the nose prominence gives volume to the central face and its position should be in harmony with the beauty triangle (projected cheekbones and chin). The tip should be in the line of the cheekbone prominences. The nasal dorsum should be straight or slightly concave. The best angles are: 90° angle at the tip, 110° nasolabial angle, 30° angle of nostrils to columella, 30° dorsum to profile line. The aim of Serdev Suture® techniques in beautification rhinoplasty is to improve the above-mentioned aesthetic proportions, volumes, and angles of the nose, adapted to the face as a whole. Serdev Sutures® in rhinoplasty include: tip rotation, refinement of the tip, lower and medial thirds, alar base narrowing and nasal dorsum lifting of concavities and irregularities.

Keywords: Rhinoplasty, Serdev Sutures®, nasal tip rotation, nasal tip refinement, alar base narrowing, nasal dorsum lifting, atraumatic rhinoplasty, mini-invasive, no bandages, no downtime

1. Introduction

Serdev Suture® techniques are over 20 for face (including rhinoplasty) and body liftings and/or volumizing. In rhinoplasty cases, the author used Serdev Sutures® as separate procedures or as part of complex rhinoplasties [1-17]. Their main indications are tip rotation and refinement, alar base narrowing, dorsum asymmetries and deformities, and secondary cases, where trauma is not advisable.

Earlier rhinoplasty techniques were based on closed or open operative procedures with combinations of incisions, approaches, and tip altering maneuvers, cartilage separation and their treatments, which are followed by some not very rare complications, such as tip deformation, destabilization of the nasal framework, and nasal tip support. Later, radical cartilage resections have been replaced by reshaping and reorienting of the nasal tip components. Intraoperative suture techniques of the nasal tip in open surgery became popular with McCollough and English double-dome unit procedure to increase tip projection and refinement using a horizontal mattress suture through all 4 crura just beneath the domes; with Goldman tip procedure for the wide or bulbous lobule, with Daniel domal creation suture, a horizontally placed mattress suture, which shaped each dome separately. Numerous suturing techniques appear in the literature regarding open technique rhinoplasty. All subcutaneous suture techniques listed above are used in open surgery [18-29].

Serdev Sutures® techniques represent scarless transcutaneous or transmucosal **closed approach** techniques. They could be: 1) transcutaneous methods to refine the tip or narrow the alar base; 2) transmucosal medial crura mattress sutures for tip refinement, columella sliding, and columella stabilization; 3) refinement sutures of projected lateral crura; and 4) sutures of fibrotic tissue or greater cartilages to lift depressions on the dorsum – primary or secondary. Thus, narrowing of the tip and alar base, and cartilaginous lower and medial third of the nose, etc., could be obtained. Author's needles (Figure 1) and Polycon semielastic surgical sutures guarantee the atraumatic nature of the procedure and better healing process.

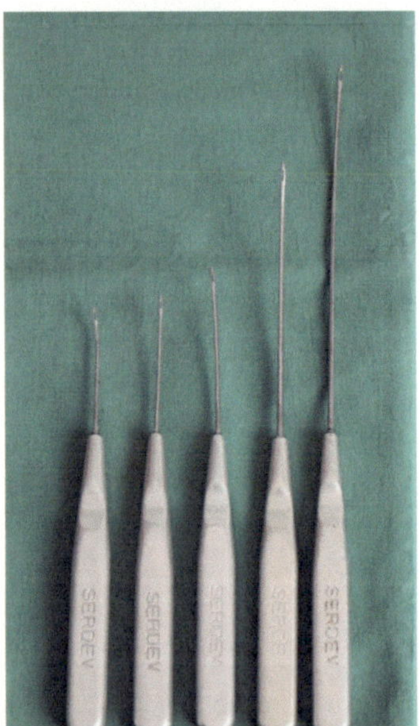

Figure 1. Curved semiblunt and semielastic Serdev® needles, with different lengths (50, 60, 80, 100, and 140 mm) and an eye at the tip.

One of the important qualities of Serdev® needles is that they create a round skin perforation point and allow for easy prevention of dermis fixation during the second needle pass that completes the circle of the suture. This is an advantage over cutting needles, which create a linear skin perforation that may result in capturing dermis, and must be avoided. The result when using other needles is dimpling, which is impossible to remove.

Stable results also depend on the suture material. Thin, monofilament threads can cut through the fine nasal cartilages, especially if the latter are mobile. Polycon, braided, semielastic USP 3-0 sutures, used by the author, protect the sutured cartilages and ensure the longevity of the result.

2. Anatomy

The alar cartilages define the nasal tip. Their three crura (medial, middle, and lateral) and their junctions are of main aesthetic importance. The medial crus forms the columella and its support. Wide distance between the medial crura makes the tip look bifid or wide, depending on thin or thick soft tissue and skin. The middle crus has a lobular and a domal segment. The normal divergence angle between lobular segments should be close to 30°. Both divergence and domal angle can form a wide tip. The length of the lobular segment is also responsible for the tip shape.

2.1. Indications for nasal tip, medial and lower third refinement via Serdev Sutures®

Indications are specific wide tip deformities: bifid tip with a dimple between the two tips, bulbous tip with flat domal segment and broad convex lateral crura; boxy tip with rectangular shape; ball tip with alar cartilages, which are too large and convex; bulky tip with thick skin, too heavy in comparison to the rest of the nose.

3. Tip rotation and dorsal alienation

3.1. Transcutaneous suture for lifting of all 4 crura or only medial crura of greater alar cartilages with fixation to the periosteum of the nasal bones

Two lines of the suture are important: 1) a pass under the nasal bone periosteum, which represents the immobile fixation, and 2) a subdermal pass in the columella, holding the mobile medial crura or all 4 crura of the greater alar cartilages – their suture rotation will shorten the nose. Two connecting subdermal passes fulfill the circle of the suture. The suture dives without engaging skin in each skin perforation point (Figure 2).

3.2. Surgical technique

The needle and suture are introduced through the following planes: The pass A-B is subperiosteal (50 mm Serdev® needle is used). A1-A and B1-B are subdermal connecting passed (60 mm Serdev® needle is used). The tip fixation pass A1-B1 is subdermal and fixes the greater alar cartilages. The knot could be placed in any point and should over-rotate the tip with about 2 mm (Figures 2 and 3). Skilled surgeons can change the A1-B1 pass, using only one perforation point in the middle of the columella just below the dome (point C) and make sure to pass subdermally and fix the greater alar cartilages.

Video: http://www.youtube.com/watch?v=nRh8NDSgDck

The same tip rotation is possible if only the medial crura of the greater alar cartilages are fixed just below the dome. This technique requires contamination prevention. The passes should not perforate into the nostrils.

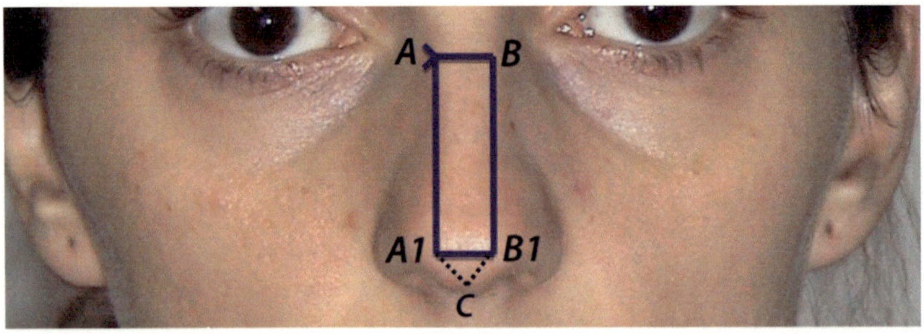

Figure 2. Tip rotation by transcutaneous suture: Pass A1-B1 should be subdermal to hold and rotate the greater alar cartilages and fix them to the subperiosteal A-B pass of the suture.

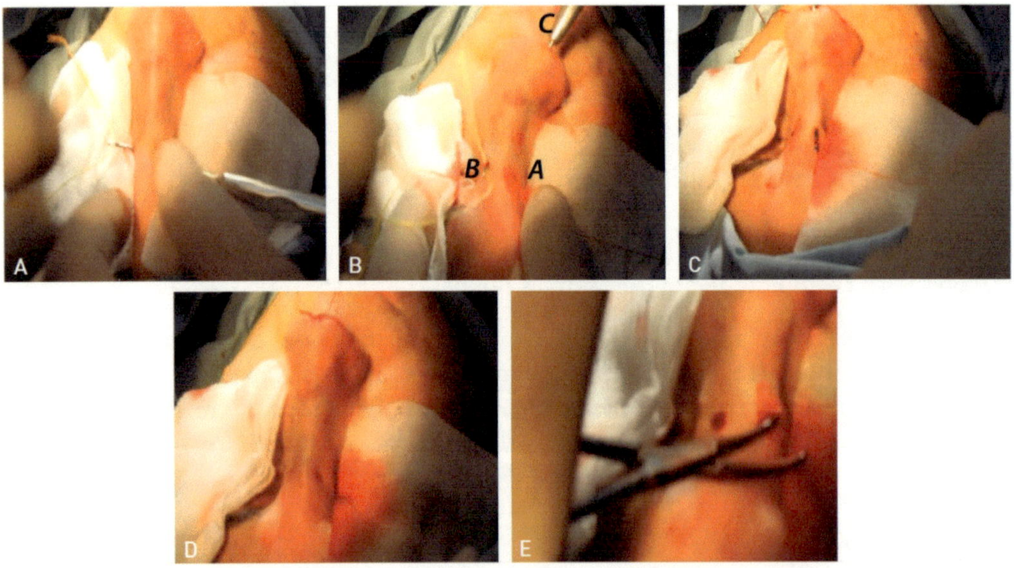

Figure 3. Nasal tip rotation by suspension of the greater alar cartilages to the nasal bone, **A.** Needle perforation through the nasal bone periosteum. The needle is loaded and the suture will be introduced in line B-A subperiosteally.

B. Using one skin perforation point in the middle of the columella, just below the dome, the first connecting needle pass is done to lift the left greater alar cartilage dome with fixation to the nasal bone periosteum. The needle reaches the left-side skin perforation point B at the level of the subperiosteal pass. The needle is loaded and the suture will be introduced in line B-C subdermally **C.** Using the same skin perforation point in the middle of the columella, just below the dome, the second connecting needle pass is done to lift the right greater alar cartilage dome with fixation to the nasal bone periosteum. The needle reaches the right side skin perforation point A at the level of the subperiosteal pass. The needle is loaded and the suture will be introduced in line A-C subdermally **D.** Suture is tied to slightly overcorrect the position of the nasal tip. E. Removal of skin dimples with a mosquito clamp – http://www.youtube.com/watch?v=nRh8NDSgDck

Nasal tip rotation by suture is mostly useful in Asians and Afro-Americans, having softer septum and unstable columella. In Caucasians with a hard septum the tip could not be lifted by suture and we perform another technique of the author – the T-excision and columella sliding, which could be supported by suture if necessary. The tip rotation suture is very helpful to align the dorsum, especially in irregular dorsum and secondary rhinoplasties.

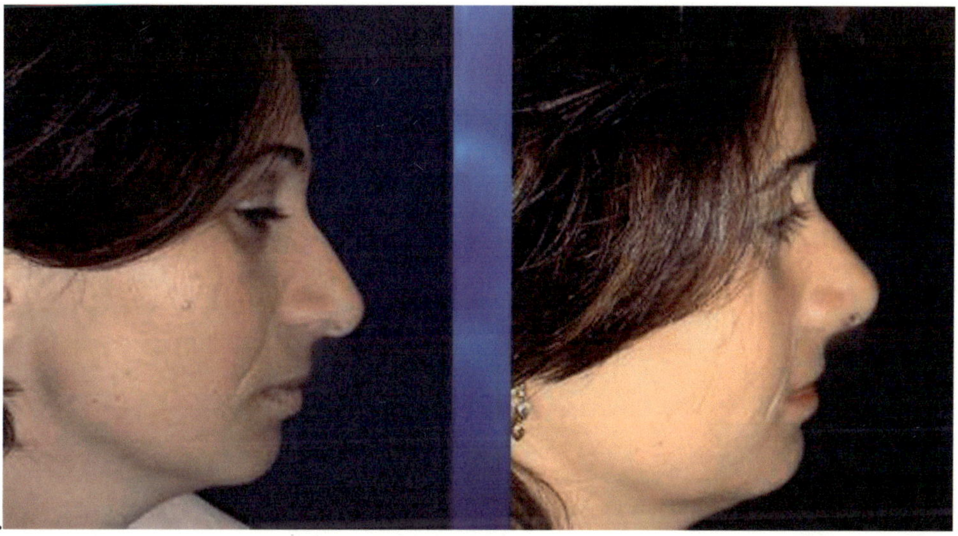

A. B.

Figure 4. Nasal tip rotation via Serdev Suture® in a Caucasian patient. **A.** Before. **B.** After. Suture lift is possible if the long nose has a soft septum of normal length, and the elongation is represented by elongated mucosa.

4. Tip refinement

4.1. Tip refinement using transcutaneous transdomal suture of all 4 crura

A 50 mm curved semielastic Serdev® needle and semielastic Polycon sutures USP 3-0 are preferred for these specific delicate cartilages. They have prolonged absorption (2 years, i.e., after final fibrosis is obtained and foreign materials are no more necessary). Rigid and thin threads can perform like scalpels and cut through cartilages.

Nonabsorbable sutures are potential foreign bodies for late complications (infection, foreign body reaction, and extrusion). Early absorbable suture material disappears sooner than needed.

Author's transcutaneous sutures do not engage skin. The direct contact between cartilage surfaces in suture techniques stimulates fibrotic formation, which guarantees the stability of the result.

There is a selection of variation in each technique, modifications or combinations of techniques. For tip refinement, the author mostly uses the transdomal technique of suturing all 4 crura.

This method is very effective for narrowing the tip. It could be also used to additionally increase the tip projection. Skin perforation points are usually positioned the level of the tip point on either side, to insert a horizontal mattress suture through all 4 crura subdomally. It is a double dome suture (Figure 5) to narrow the tip by bringing the domes together.

4.1.1. Surgical technique

The transdomal suture uses 2 skin punctures and consists of 2 needle passes, without engaging skin. Each needle pass uses a different but parallel path through the cartilages. The transcutaneous suture is diving, buried below the skin. It attaches only cartilages, without including dermis in the suture. Skin and its perforations can be moved up and down the cartilages to obtain a distance of 2–3 mm between the parallel passes. Both needle passes have to be placed in the domal area without perforating the nostril in order to prevent contamination and compromising the result. The suture could be placed 3–4 mm posterior to the dome, to preserve the separation between the domes in front. The knots should be tied under elastic tension.

4.1.2. Clinical cases

The transcutaneous transdomal suture could be applied as a separate technique or as a part of primary or secondary rhinoplasty. It is simpler and safer than subcutaneous sutures in open rhinoplasty and their sequellae. It closes the divergence and dome angles atraumatically, thus saving time during operation, and shortens recovery.

4.2. Tip refinement using transmucosal domal suture of medial crura

This method is usually combined with the author's closed rhinoplasty techniques, such as T-excision and columella sliding. The suture should be placed as high as possible to fix the domal medial crura. There is no need for this suture to be buried below the nasal mucosa, which is involved on each side in the transmucosal mattress suture. Using absorbable sutures, the fibrosis stabilizes the effect after the first 3–4 weeks. If suture is not absorbable, it has to be removed after 3 weeks.

Medial crural fixation suture is used to fix the medial crura and to close the divergence angle between lobular segments of medial crura. This suture can refine the tip in cases of an open divergence angle of medial crura and normal domal angle. If the domal angle is more open, then the medial crura fixation suture can be an additional correction. The suture gathers the

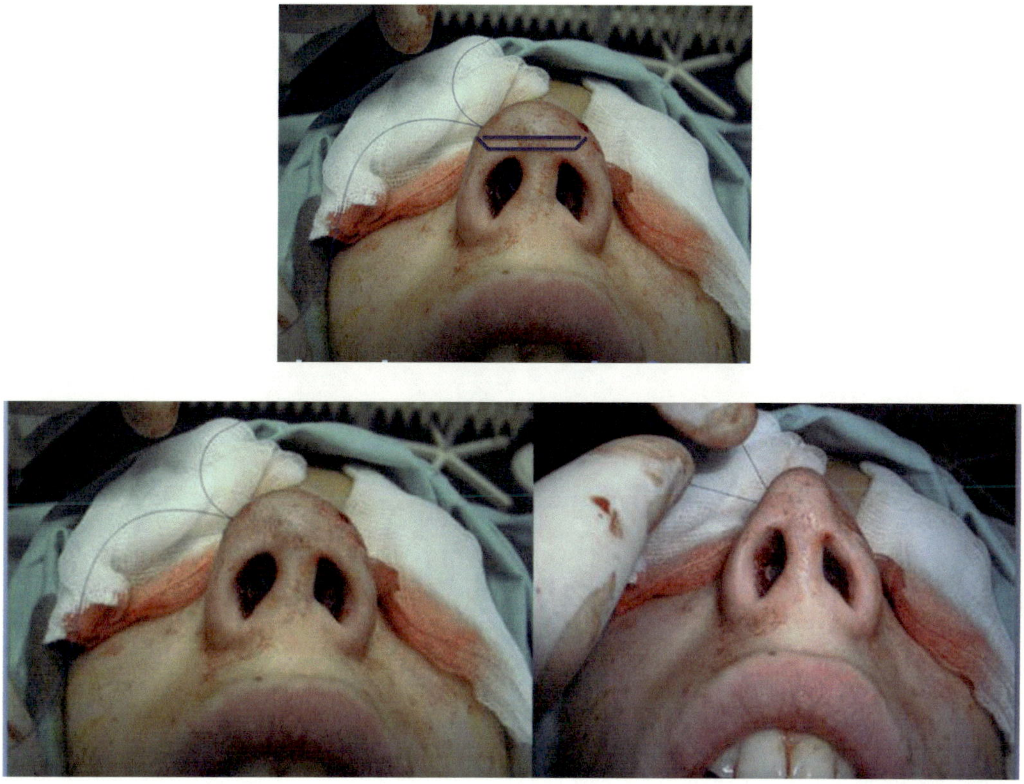

Figure 5. Transcutaneous transdomal suture of all 4 crura. The suture is made through the domal part of the lower alar cartilages. The tip deviation on the photo is due to the traction during knotting of the suture. The distance between the passes should be 2–3 mm. The suture should be placed in the domal tissue only. Be careful not to enter through the nostril as this will cause suture contamination. Dermis should not be engaged in order to prevent from dimples. Dimpling will be removed using a mosquito instrument.

A. 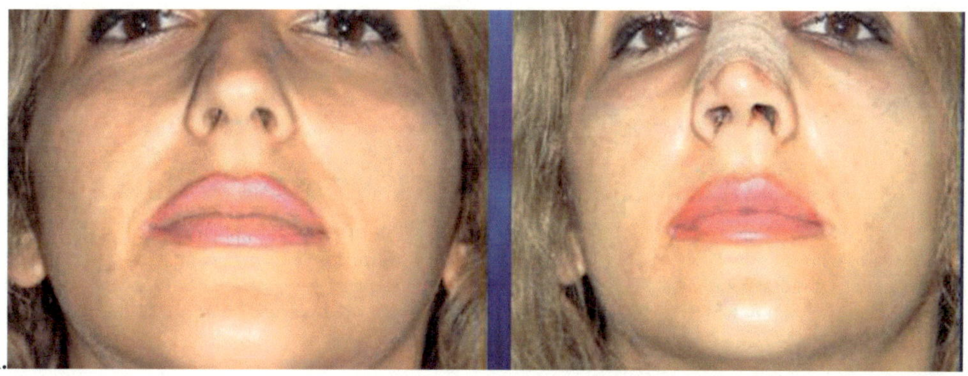 B.

Figure 6. A. Before. Aquiline nose with a wide dome. **B.** After. Day 1 after rhinoplasty: T-excision, humpectomy, digital fracture, columella sliding, and tip refinement using transcutaneous suture.

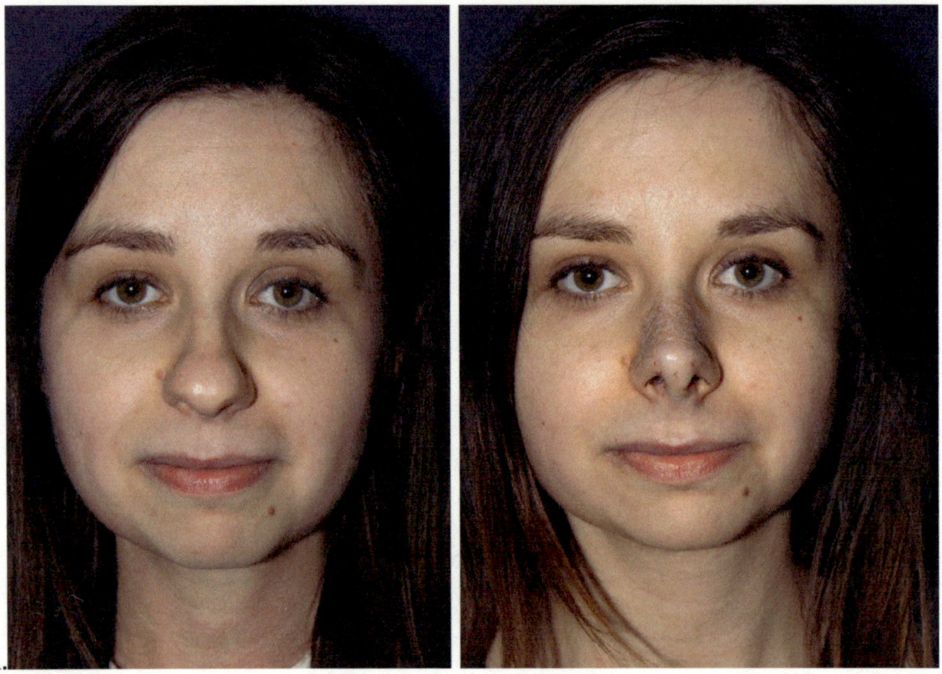

A. B.

Figure 7. A. Before. Aquiline nose with a bulbous tip and hanging columella. Wide volume at the tip, disrupting the beauty triangle and the proportions of the face. **B.** Day 1 after T-excision, humpectomy, digital fracture, columella sliding, and two transcutaneous transdomal sutures for nasal tip and nasal lower third refinement, and transmucosal domal suture to stabilize dome refinement (See Section 6.2.2.). A case with no bruising, due to the atraumatic nature of the techniques. Narrow tip and dorsum, as well as better proportions of the face are present.

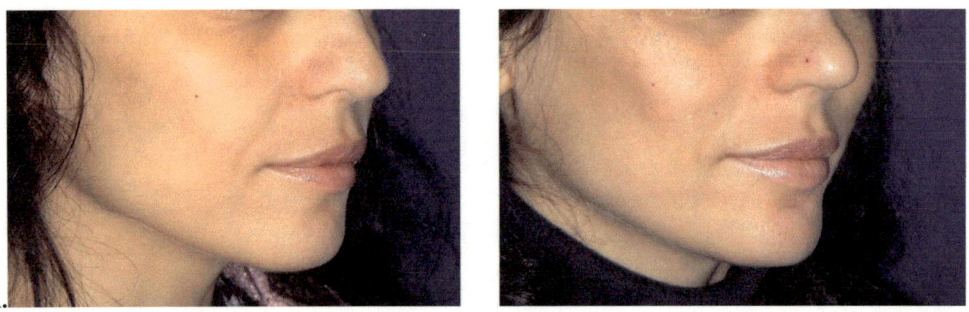

A. B.

Figure 8. A. Before. Long nose. **B.** After. Day 1 after T-excision for tip rotation and transcutaneous transdomal suture for tip refinement. Simultaneous cheekbone lifting and chin enhancement using Serdev Sutures®. A small crust is present at the perforation point. Swelling is present. The patient – TV reporter has used makeup on her way to work.

open medial crura and gives additional projection to the domes. A horizontal mattress suture is placed through mucosa and both medial crura (Figure 9). The domal symmetry can be adjusted with the position of the needle perforating both medial crura. If there is asymmetry of both tips, the needle pass through cartilages should be parallel to the asymmetric defining points of the tip to keep symmetry in the tip area (Figure 1, Chapter 5).

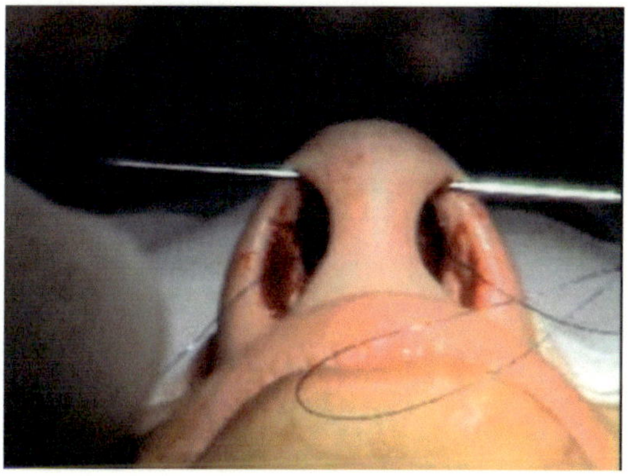

Figure 9. Transmucosal domal suture of medial crura for tip refinement, parallel to the tip defining points.

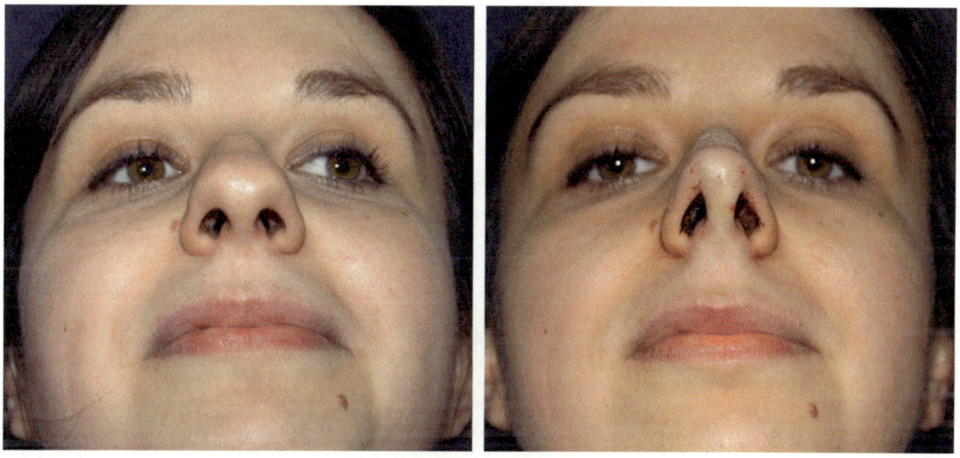

Figure 10. A. Before. A case of aquiline nose with a bulbous tip. **B.** Transcutaneous transdomal and transmucosal domal suture for tip refinement. Day 1 after simultaneous T-excision, humpectomy, digital fracture, columella sliding, two transcutaneous transdomal sutures for nasal tip and nasal lower third refinement, and transmucosal domal suture to stabilize dome refinement.

If both sides of the tip are not equal in projection, a domal equalization of symmetry may need an additional nonhorizontal transdomal or medial crura suture.

Both suture types give good refining definition and at the same time a projection effect. In cases of bulbous tip, transdermal suture of all 4 crura is preferable. Both sutures can be used separately, combined, or as a part of a complex rhinoplasty.

5. Refinement of the dorsum

5.1. Refinement of nasal lower third using lateral crura transcutaneous suspension suture

If prominent lateral crura widen the lower third of the nose, then spanning sutures are used by the author to reduce their convexity and narrow the area cephalic to the tip. The transcutaneous suture should be placed at the highest convexity area, in order to suppress it. Fixation of the suture to a higher point of the dorsal septum is used in selected cases to additionally rotate the tip.

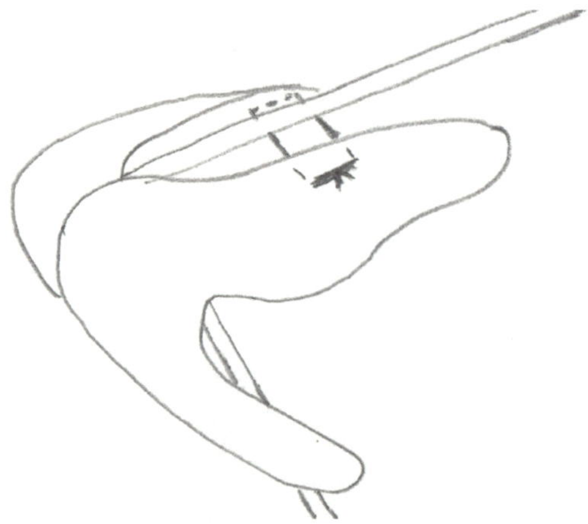

Figure 11. Transcutaneous suspension suture of the lateral crura of the greater alar cartilages for nasal lower third refinement.

A.

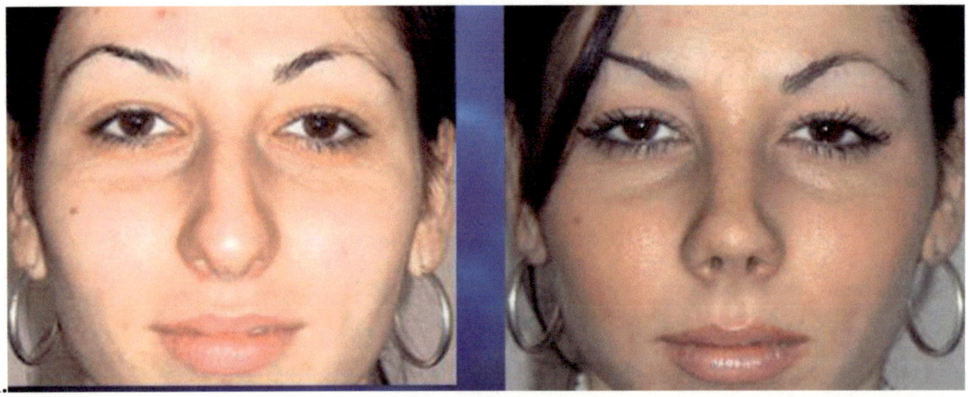

B.

Figure 12. A. Before. Slightly deviated aquiline long nose. No septal deviation is present, only nasal bone irregularity. Bulbous tip with hanging columella. **B.** After. Simultaneous T-excision, humpectomy, digital fracture to straighten the nasal pyramid, columella sliding, transcutaneous transdomal suture for tip refinement, and transcutaneous suspension suture of the lateral crura of the greater alar cartilages for lower nasal third refinement.

http://dx.doi.org/10.5772/62074

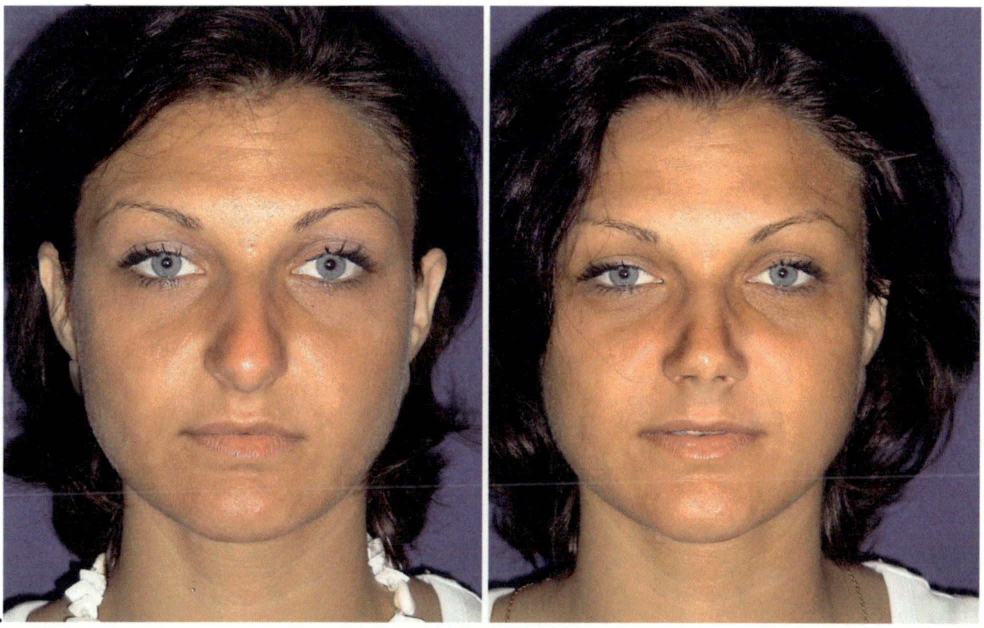

A. B.

Figure 13. A. Before. **B.** After simultaneous T-excision for nasal tip rotation, columella sliding for tip projection, transcutaneous transdomal suture for tip refinement and transcutaneous suspension suture of the lateral crura of the greater alar cartilages for lower nasal third refinement.

5.2. Refinement of nasal medial third using transcutaneous suture of upper lateral cartilages

This suture (author's) is useful in primary cases with wide upper lateral cartilages or mostly in secondary cases with open cartilage and bony roof after humpectomy.

In secondary cases, digital fracture of the nasal bones and sutures of upper lateral cartilages are used by the author to optimally close the open roof, project and narrow the dorsum at the nasal medial third. One or more transcutaneous sutures could be placed along the cartilage part of the nose at the medial third, lower third, and the tip of the nose for whole dorsum refinement (Figure 14). Fixation of the suture to the dorsal septum is used in selected cases for stabilization, if necessary.

This maneuver is easy, catching the dorsal septum with the semiblunt, semielastic, curved Serdev® needles. They create a round skin perforation point and allow for easy prevention of dermis fixation during the second needle pass. This is an advantage over cutting needles, which create a linear skin perforation that in most cases leads to fixation of the dermis – the result is dimpling, which is impossible to remove.

Stable results also depend on the suture material. Thin, monofilament threads can cut through the fine cartilages. Polycon sutures, braided, semielastic, USP 3-0 protect the sutured cartilages and ensure longevity of the result.

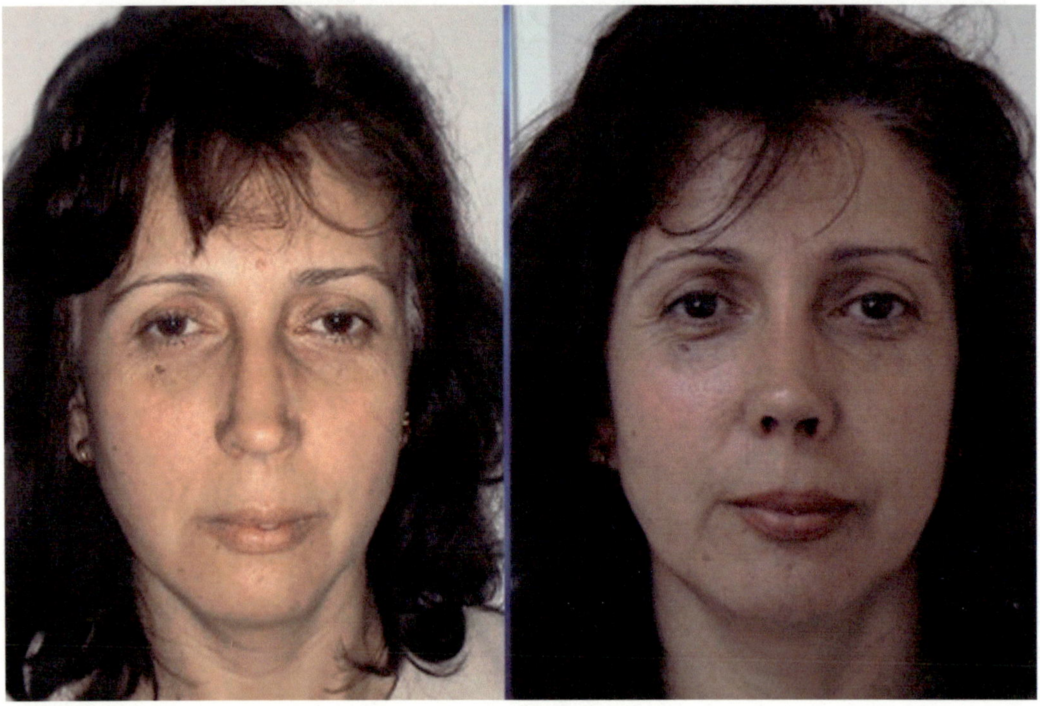

Figure 14. A case with serial sutures along the dorsum to achieve refinement.

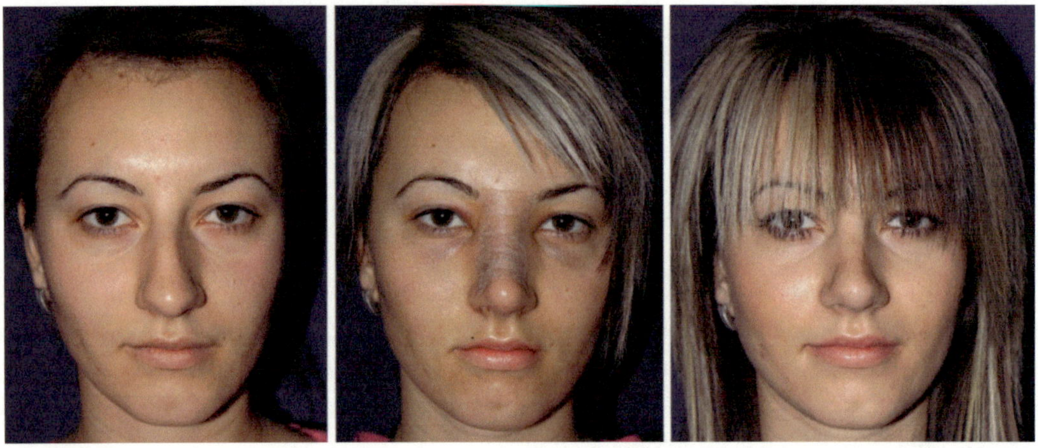

Figure 15. Before, 3 days, and 2 months after T-excision, humpectomy, digital fracture for alignment, and sutures for tip and lower nasal third refinement.

http://dx.doi.org/10.5772/62074

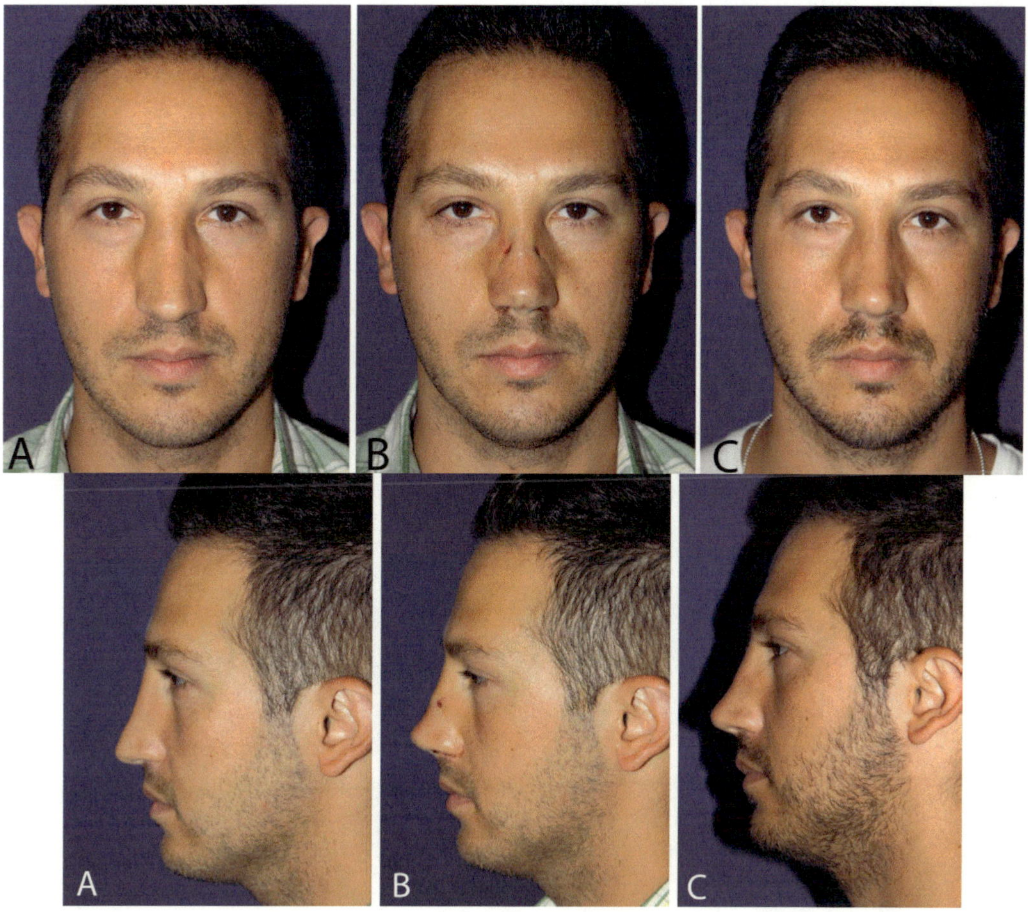

Figure 16. Secondary case. A third rhinoplasty procedure could offer a lot of complications. A. Before. Flat nose, very wide step form base of the nasal bones after lateral osteotomy. **B.** Immediate result after T-excision for nasal tip rotation, columella sliding for tip projection, and transcutaneous suture of the upper lateral cartilages for narrowing, reforming and lifting/projection of the nasal dorsum. Better angles of the nose and proportions of the face. **C.** 3 months later. The nose is proportional, with much better and nearly normal "nonoperated appearance" after atraumatic mini-invasive surgery.

6. Alar base narrowing

The aesthetic angle of the nostrils between the columella and lateral alae should be 30°. Wide alar base with ethnic unstable columella in Asian, Afro-American, and Latino-American patients could need additional columella stabilization suture and transdomal suture for tip refinement.

Alar base narrowing has the additional effect of tip projection.

Deviations and deformities in cases of wide alar base could be different, depending on ethnos, protruding medial crura, deviated nasal spine, etc. (Figure 17A, B, C). Resection and excision techniques are well known and applicable. In numerous cases the author meets patients who reject excisions and scars, and prefer his suture techniques.

The suture technique represents 2 parallel passes (1–2 mm distance between them), using 2 skin punctures at both nasolabial angles narrowing both nostrils (Figure 17A), or unilateral in cases of one medial crus protruding end (Figure. 17B), or narrowing only the divergent medial crura or combination of sutures (Figure 17 C, D). Suture lines should pass subdermally, exactly caudal to the nostrils and nasal spine. (**NB:** Do not perforate into the nostrils, in order to avoid contamination.)

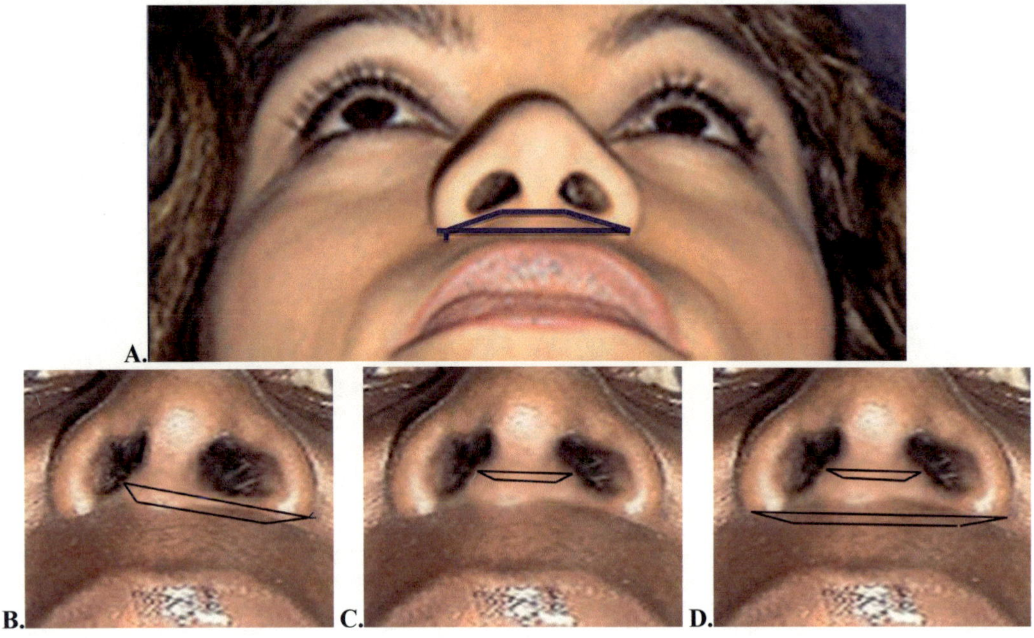

Figure 17. A. If the wide alar base is symmetrical, the suture represents 2 parallel passes (1–2 mm distance between them), using 2 skin punctures at both nasolabial angles. The suture lines should pass subdermally, exactly caudal to the nostrils and nasal spine. **B.** If the alar base is asymmetrical due to protruding end of one medial crus, the suture can be unilateral, or a combination of A and B. **C.** If the columella is wide due to divergent footplates of the medial crura of greater alar cartilages, the suture can fix only them. **D.** If a combination of deviations and deformities are present, different sutures can be used simultaneously.

If the wide alar base is symmetrical, the suture represents 2 parallel passes (1–2 mm distance between them), using 2 skin punctures at both nasolabial angles. Suture lines should pass subdermally, exactly caudal to nostrils and nasal spine (Figure 17A).

There are cases of wide alar base with asymmetrical columella due to one-side divergent medial crus footplate. Then the suture can be unilateral (Figure 17B) or a combination (Figure 17A and B). If the columella is wide due to very divergent footplates of medial crura, the suture can fix only the divergent end of columella, or any combination of the sutures above, including tip refinement.

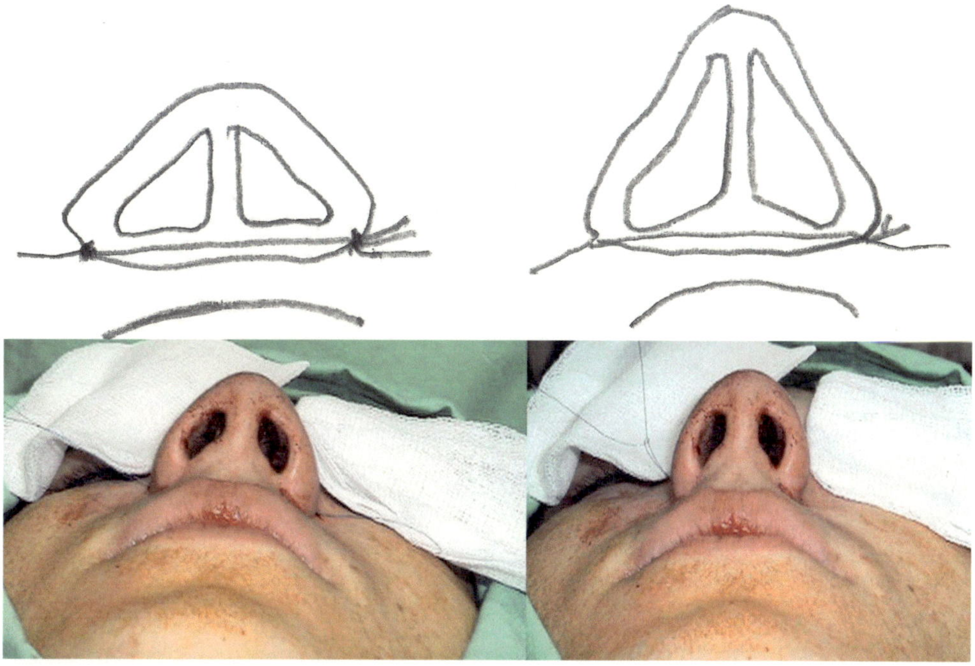

Figure 18. The suture for alar base refinement should obtain the 30° angle of the nostrils at the tip. If not possible, additional tip refinement should be performed.

A.

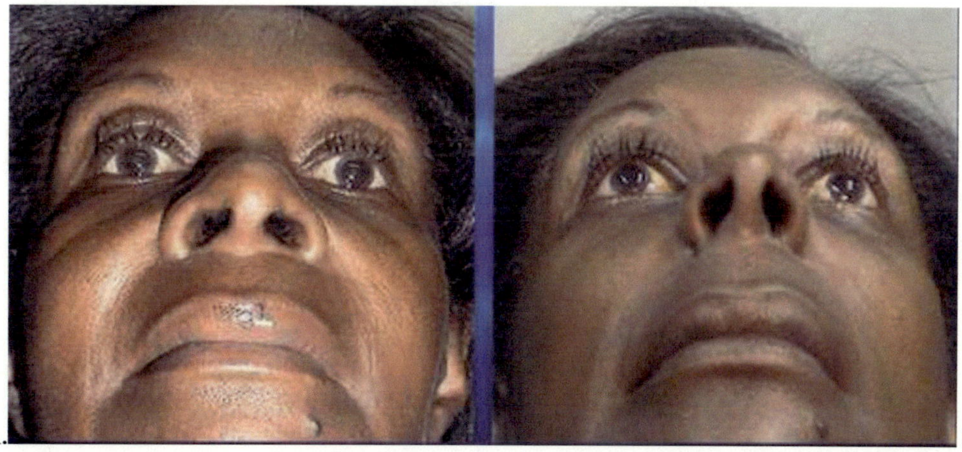

B.

Figure 19. A Before and **B.** After alar base narrowing in Afro-American patient. Good tip projection and alar angle at the tip.

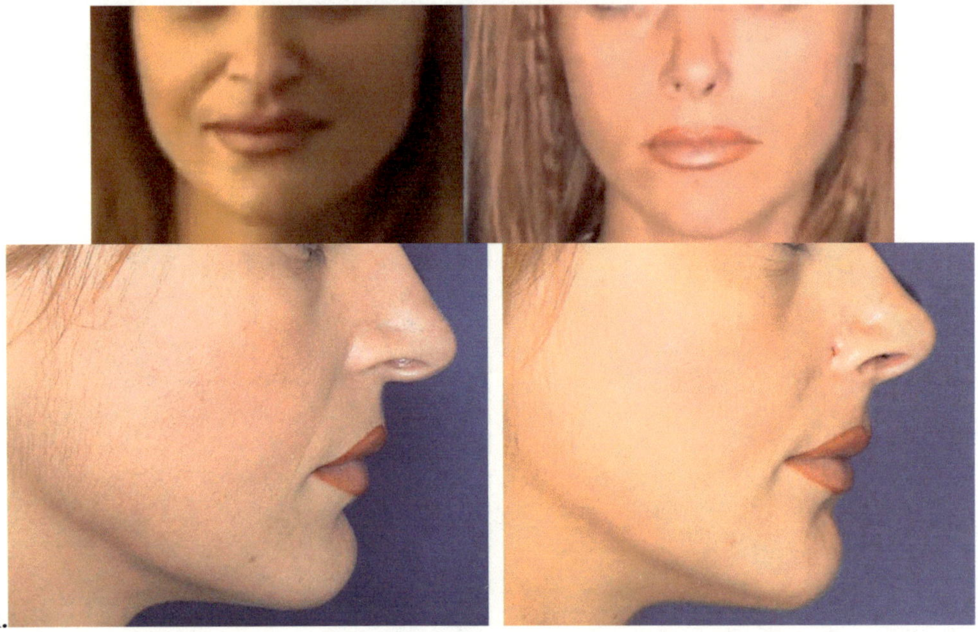

A. B.

Figure 20. A. Before. Long nose with asymmetric nostrils. **B.** After T-excision for tip rotation and unilateral narrowing of the alar base. Photo is taken immediately after the operation.

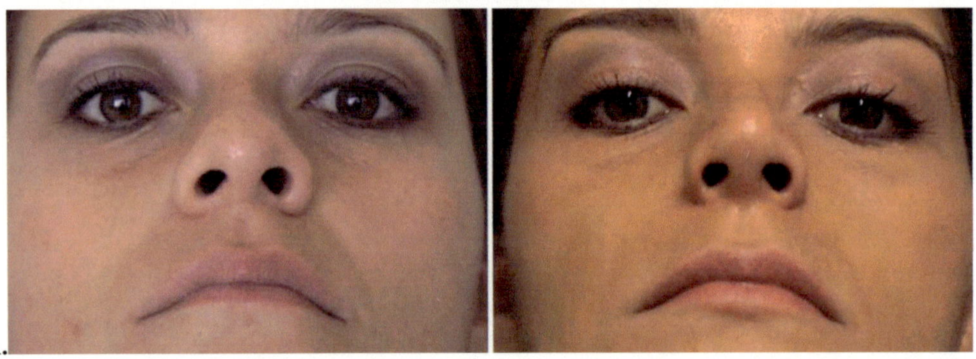

A. B.

Figure 21. A case of tip refinement and alar base narrowing by sutures in Latino-American patient. Additional brow lift suture has been performed simultaneously.

Serdev Suture® techniques in rhinoplasty have multiple modifications, they are time-saving, prevent trauma, with immediate results, and no downtime. The post-op period is short. There is no bruising; immediate or prompt return to work and social life. No bandages or tampons are necessary.

Alar base narrowing is a very important type of Caucasian-type beautification in Afro-Americans and Asians. It provides refinement in Caucasian faces.

http://dx.doi.org/10.5772/62074

7. Sutures for dorsum prominence

7.1. In primary and secondary depressions and concavities

The author's transcutaneous sutures are placed just above the nasal bones and cartilages to fix fibrotic tissue, in order to project the soft tissue and skin. The dorsal part of cartilages could be sutured as well. A fixation of cartilages to the septum in primary and secondary open roof cases can be used for this purpose as well. In addition, these sutures narrow the nasal dorsum.

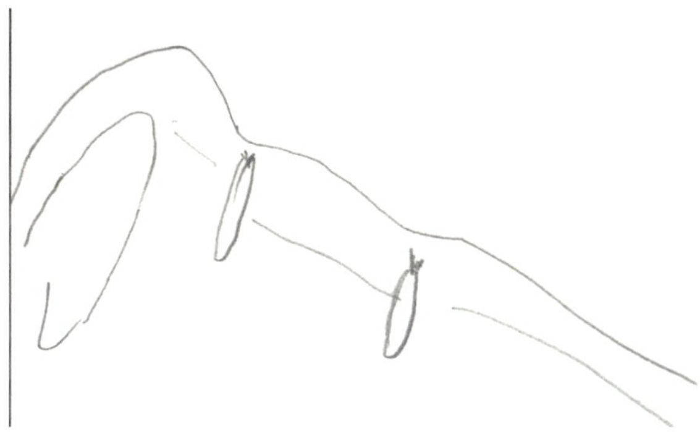

Figure 22. Serdev Sutures® for lifting of nasal dorsum in cases of concavities, and primary and secondary defects.

A. 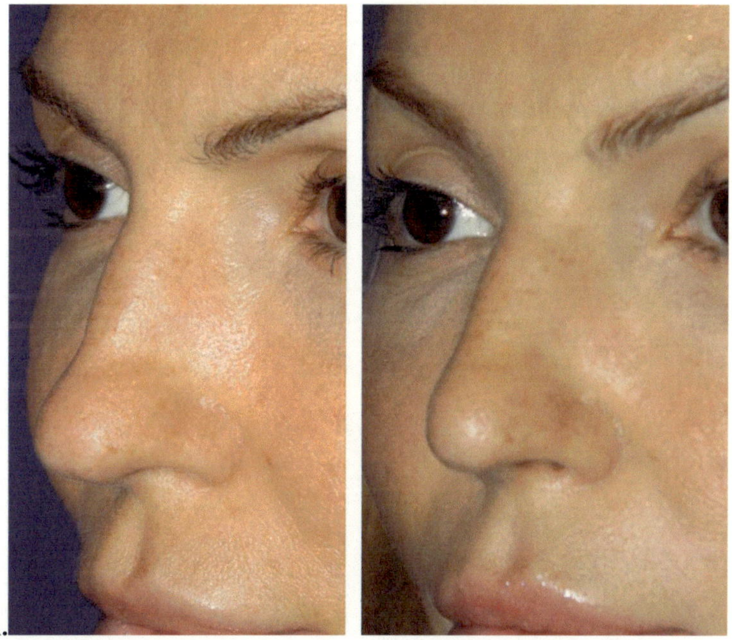 B.

Figure 23. Serdev Suture® for dorsum alignment in supratip depression.

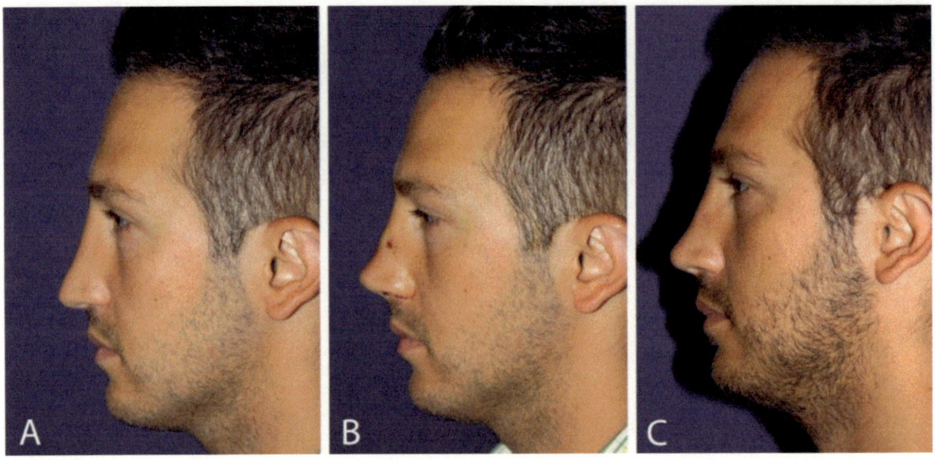

Figure 24. Serdev Suture® for lifting of the dorsum in a secondary open roof case with flat nasal appearance and T-excision for correction of the long nose and achieving of appropriate aesthetic proportions, volumes, and angles.

8. Conclusion

Serdev Sutures® in rhinoplasty, as mini-invasive and atraumatic procedures, used separately or as part of complex rhinoplasty, show advantages over other rhinoplasty techniques. Author's techniques are time-saving, atraumatic operations with great results and complication rate lower than 0.003% [1-3]. Transcutaneous suture techniques have advantages over medical rhinoplasty using temporary fillers as well, because the time of procedure is the same or shorter, but the result is permanent.

Author details

Nikolay P. Serdev*

Address all correspondence to: serdev@gmail.com

New Bulgarian University, Sofia, Medical Centre "Aesthetic Surgery and Aesthetic Medicine," Sofia, Bulgaria

References

[1] Serdev NP. Suture Suspensions for Lifting or Volume Augmentation in Face and Body (English version), 2nd Annual Meeting of the National Bulgarian Society for

Aesthetic Surgery and Aesthetic Medicine, Sofia, March 18, 1994, *Int J Aesth Cosm* 2001; 1(1):2561-2568

[2] Serdev NP. Principles of Face Beautification, Third World Congress of the International Society of Aesthetic Surgery, Tokyo April 8-10, 2000, 9W58

[3] Serdev NP. Course: Beautification rhinoplasty, t-zone excision, columella sliding, suture methods, Updates in IV sedation and analgesia. 2005; Feb 23. Available from: http://ijcs.org/courses/2005/90/index.php

[4] Serdev NP. Serdev sutures for: Nasal tip refinement, nasal tip rotation, Nasal alar base narrowing. *Int J Cosm Surg* 2007; 7(1):328- 386

[5] Serdev NP. Serdev techniques in beautification rhinoplasty: T-zone excision, columella sliding, Serdev sutures. *Int J Cosm Surg* 2008; 8(1):388-469

[6] Serdev NP. Nasal tip refinement, rotation, projection, alar base narrowing In: Serdev NP, Ed. *Serdev Sutures® Face and Body Lifts and/or Volumising*. Marllor editions, Italy, 2013: 75-81

[7] Serdev NP. Serdev Sutures® in middle face 4. Beautification rhinoplasty – tip rotation and refinement, alar base narrowing. In: Serdev NP, Ed. *Miniinvasive Face and Body Lifts – Closed Suture Lifts or Barded Thread Lifts*. Intech, Rijeka, 2013. Available from http://www.intechopen.com/books/miniinvasive-face-and-body-lifts-closed-suture-lifts-or-barbed-thread-lifts/serdev-sutures-in-middle-face.

[8] Serdev NP. Chin enhancement by scarless Serdev suture and Serdev rhinoplasty without tampons and bandages. Shop the world for beauty secrets E5 (Video) YouTube 2009; 12.05. Available from http://www.youtube.com/watch?v=2wj5q3RCvuQ.

[9] Serdev NP. Secondary rhinoplasty - Tip rotation by Serdev suture after hump removal (video) YouTube 2011; 12.04. Available from http://www.youtube.com/watch?v=nRh8NDSgDck

[10] Serdev NP. Rhinoplasty bloodless beautification in minutes, no bruising, no tampons, no plaster 19.02.2014 http://www.youtube.com/watch?v=pRSGBqe8r6E

[11] Serdev NP. Rhinoplasty Dr Serdev author methods 1.07.2009 http://www.youtube.com/watch?v=Ci53JRQlJFc

[12] Serdev NP. Nasal tip rotation by Serdev suture in secondary rhinoplasty 31.05.2012 http://www.youtube.com/watch?v=IClFcRur-gs

[13] Serdev NP. Beautification rhinoplasty, T-excision, columella sliding, 6.04.2009 http://www.youtube.com/watch?v=xe6lA-3fY6c

[14] Serdev NP. Beautification rhinoplasty in a long nose t excision columella sliding 26.10.2013 г. http://www.youtube.com/watch?v=v1wMYoOayKc

[15] Serdev NP. Simultaneous brow lift by Serdev suture with chin dimple and secondary rhinoplasty 7.04.2009. http://www.youtube.com/watch?v=jWQocHglFWs

[16] Serdev NP. Rhinoplasty. Tip refinement by Serdev suture. No scars, 27.01.2010 r. http://www.youtube.com/watch?v=o2Ypkxqes7w

[17] Serdev NP. Live on TV Rhinoplasty, Brow Suture Lift, Chin Enhancement 10.01.2013 r. http://www.youtube.com/watch?v=H73PTB2xyKU

[18] Behmand RA, Ghavami A, Guyuron B. Nasal tip sutures, part I: the evolution. *Plast Reconstr Surg* 2003;112(4):1125-1129, discussion 1146-1149.

[19] Tebbetts JB. Shaping and positioning the nasal tip without structural disruption: a new, systematic approach. *Plast Reconstr Surg* 1994;94(1):61-77.

[20] Mocella S, Bianchi N. Double interdomal suture in nasal tip sculpturing. *Facial Plast Surg* 1997;13(3):179-196

[21] . Suture contouring of the nasal tip. *Arch Facial Plast Surg* 2000;2(1): 34-42.

[22] Leach JL, Athre RS. Four suture tip rhinoplasty: a powerful tool for controlling tip dynamics. *Otolaryngol Head Neck Surg* 2006;135(2):227-231.

[23] Tardy ME, Cheng E. Transdomal suture refinement of the nasal tip. *Facial Plast Surg* 1987;4(4):317-326.

[24] Papel ID. Interlocked transdomal suture technique for the wide interdomal space in rhinoplasty. *Arch Facial Plast Surg* 2005;7(6):414-417.

[25] Daniel RK. Rhinoplasty: a simplified, three-stitch, open tip suture technique, part I: primary rhinoplasty. *Plast Reconstr Surg* 1999;103(5):1491-1502.

[26] McCollough EG, English JL. A new twist in nasal tip surgery: an alternative to the Goldman tip for the wide or bulbous lobule. *Arch Otolaryngol* 1985;111 (8):524-529.

[27] Daniel RK. Rhinoplasty: creating an aesthetic tip: a preliminary report. *Plast Reconstr Surg* 1987;80(6):775-783.

[28] Kridel RW, Konior FJ, Shumrick KA, Wright WK. Advances in nasal tip surgery: the lateral crural steal. *Arch Otolaryngol Head Neck Surg* 1989;115(10):1206-1212.

[29] Pastorek NJ, Becker DG. Treating the caudal septal deflection. *Arch Facial Plast Surg* 2000;2(3):217-220.

[30] Gruber RP, Friedman GD. Suture algorithm for the broad or bulbous nasal tip. *Plast Reconstr Surg* 2002;110(7):1752-1764, discussion 1765-1768.

Chapter 7

Depressor Septi Nasi Muscle Resection or Nerve Block

Daniel G. Moina and Gabriel M. Moina

Additional information is available at the end of the chapter

http://dx.doi.org/10.5772/62073

Abstract

In our daily practice, we usually perform the rhinoplasty without considering the dynamic functions.The depressor septi nasi muscle (DSNM) is very important in nose dynamics. Its hyperactivity in some rhinoplasty patients while they smiling or speaking causes a deformity that includes drooping of the nasal tip, elevation and shortening of the upper lip, and increased maxillary gingival show. The dissection of the depressor septi muscle during rhinoplasty can improve the tip-upper lip relationship in appropriately selected patients.

To manage this functional part of rhinoplasty, we aimed to clarify the anatomic study, surgical indications, rationale for the operative technique, and clinical cases are presented.

Keywords: Depressor septi nasi muscle, Nasalis muscle, Nose muscle, Nasal tip drooping, Nose tip Fall, Smile test, Open rhinoplasty, Close rhinoplasty, nasolabial complex, DSNM hyperactivity, Nasal length, Facial muscles, Teeth exposure, Suspended upper lip, Gingival show, Gummy smile, Botulinum toxin, BTN-A, Nerve block

1. Introduction

1.1. Anatomy of depressor septi nasi muscle

The anatomy of the depressor septi nasi has been well studied by Rod Rohrich [1,2]. Is a small, paired muscle located on either side of the nasal septum, has four proximal attachments, footplates of the medial crura, caudal septum, dermocartilaginous ligament and anterior nasal spine, The muscle is divided by the nasal septum into bilateral and symmetric portions. On each of these portions we may observe a division in its fascicles:

- Medial: in medial position, parallel to the nasal septum.
- Intermedial: between medial and lateral.
- Lateral: this one more peripheral to the nasal septum.

They were interdigitated with the orbicularis oris. Like the other muscles of the nose is innervated by branches of the facial nerve and supplied by the facial artery.

Three variation of the depressor septi muscle were delineated (Fig.1-2):

Type I: Inserted fully into the orbicularis oris. 62 %.

Type II: Inserted into the periosteum and incompletely into the orbicularis oris. 22%.

Type III: Showed no or rudimentary depressor septi muscle. 16 %.

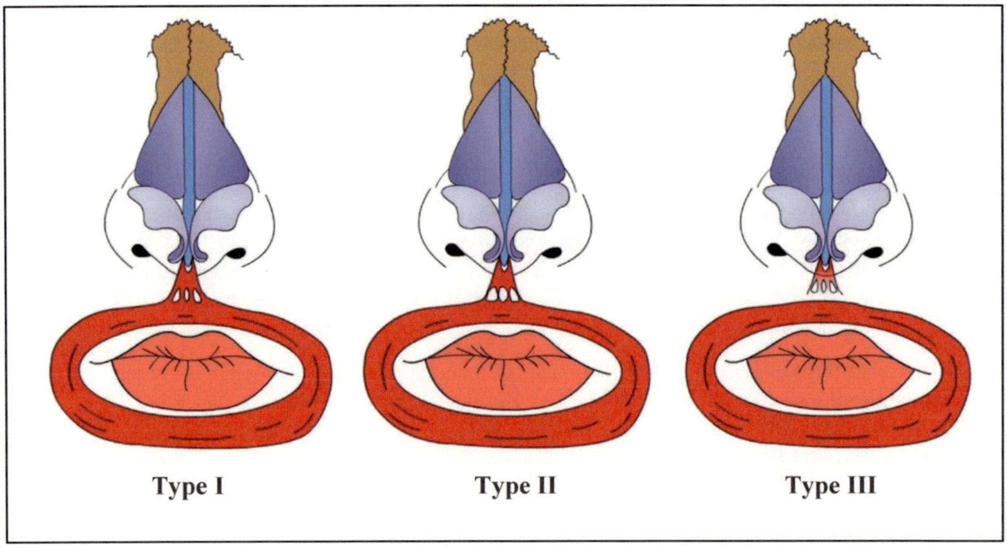

Figure 1. Anatomical variation of the depressor septi muscle.

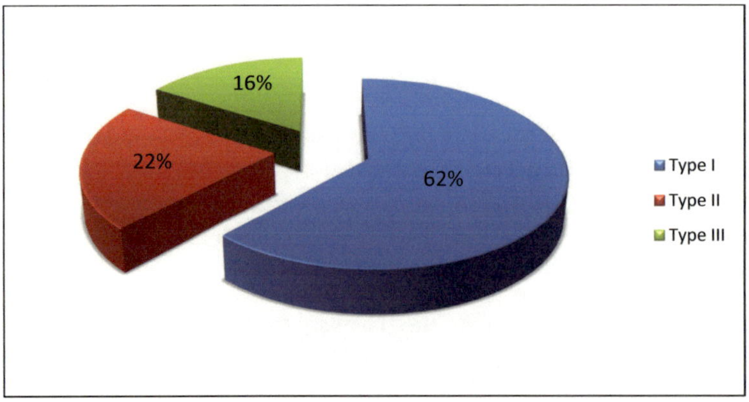

Figure 2. Percentages of anatomical variation of the depressor septi muscle.

In some patients (type I and II), animation (particularly smiling) produces a deformity characterized by:

1. A descending nasal tip.
2. A shortened upper lip.
3. An increased maxillary gingival show.
4. A transverse crease in the mid-philtral area.

In 1992 Cachay velazquez described these modifications as rhino-gingivolabial syndrome of the smile (drooping of the nasal tip, elevation and shortening of the upper lip, and increased maxillary gingival show) [3].

It's important to note that not only produces aesthetic alterations, also produces functional changes, alters the air turbulence.

The aim of treating the muscle with a minimally invasive surgery (permanent) or botulinum toxin (temporary) is decrease the effect of smiling on all four parameters.

Smile test (Wright 1976): Before the operation, during the smile analysis, front and lateral facial photographs of patients in repose and full smile were studied and at follow-up visits (Fig.3) [4,5,6].

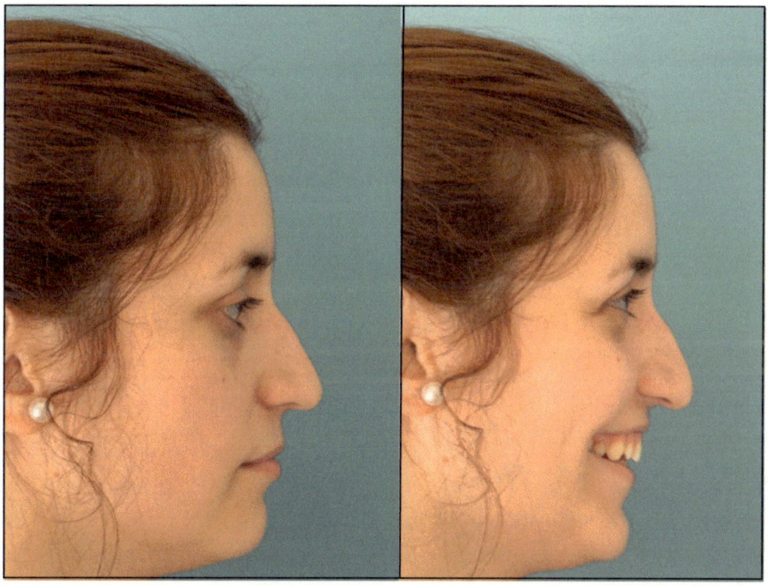

Figure 3. Smile Test, plunging of the nasal tip when smiling.

After the photographs the nasal length (NL) from the radix to the tip, tip projection (TP) from the alar-cheek junction to the tip, upper lip height (UL) and the presence or absence of a transverse upper labial crease (TC) were determined (Fig.4).

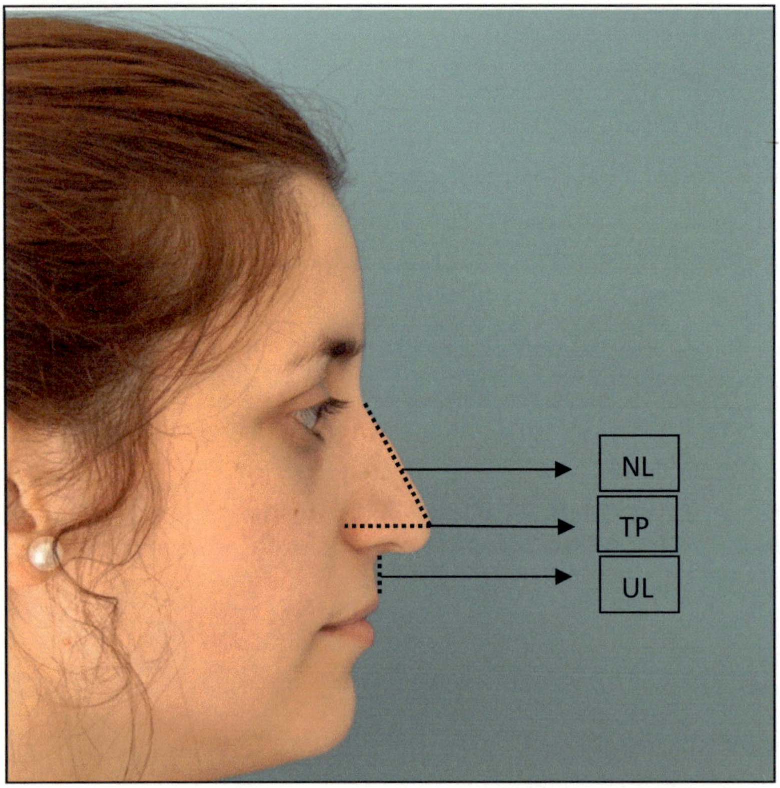

Figure 4. There main parameters used to evaluate the DSNM, NL (nasal length), TP (tip projection) and UL (upper lip height).

2. Surgical treatment of the depressor septi nasi muscle

The main and most important objective of the treatment is to remove the distal tension of the nasal tip, releasing and elevating it (Fig.5).

There are two surgical techniques for depressor septi nasi muscle treatment, transnasal and transoral technique. It's important to note that the two different techniques were not significantly different in decreasing the effects of smiling on nasal length, tip projection, upper lip height, or transverse crease.

Note: Release of this muscle also cause slight ptosis of the upper lip which may not be beneficial in patients with long upper lip.

The authors of this chapter use the transoral technique if the patient have a tethering of the frenulum and use the transnasal technique if you don't (Fig.6) [7].

http://dx.doi.org/10.5772/62073

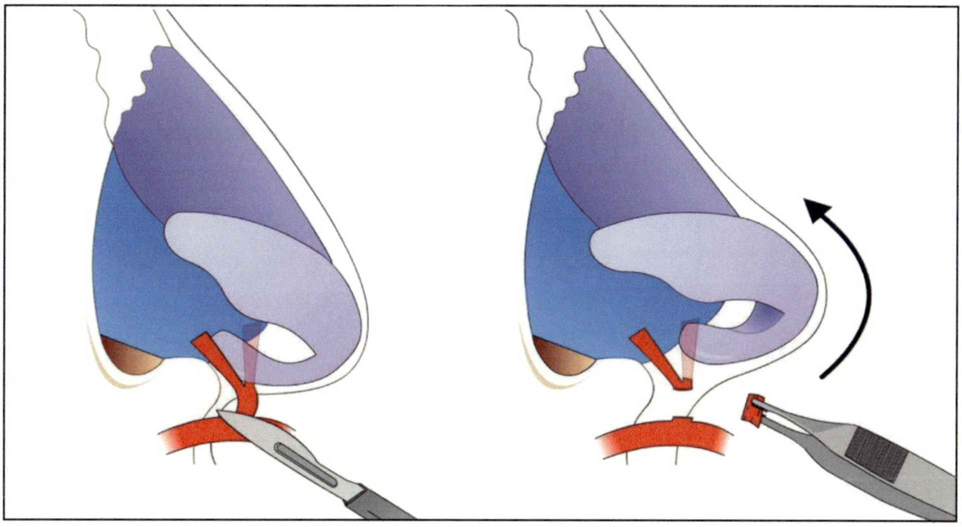

Figure 5. After resection of the muscle, the nasal tip is released.

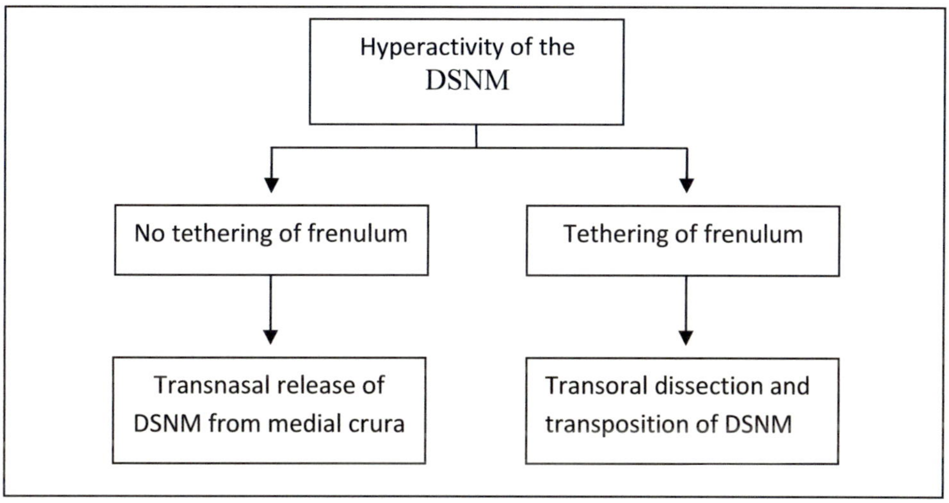

Figure 6. Algorithm for treatment of the DSNM.

- Transoral Technique (Fig.7):

We infiltrate the mucosa, frenulum and the soft tissue with 2% lidocaine with epinephrine 1:50,000, this way we produce analgesia and vasoconstriction, later on with a scalpel blade # 15 make a horizontal upper labial sulcus incision of no more than 10 mm, the depressor septi nasi muscle is released near its origin with the orbicularis oris or periosteum, transposed, and sutured to the contralateral transposed depressor septi nasi muscle (Nylon 4.0). The horizontal incision is closed vertically (vicryl 4.0).

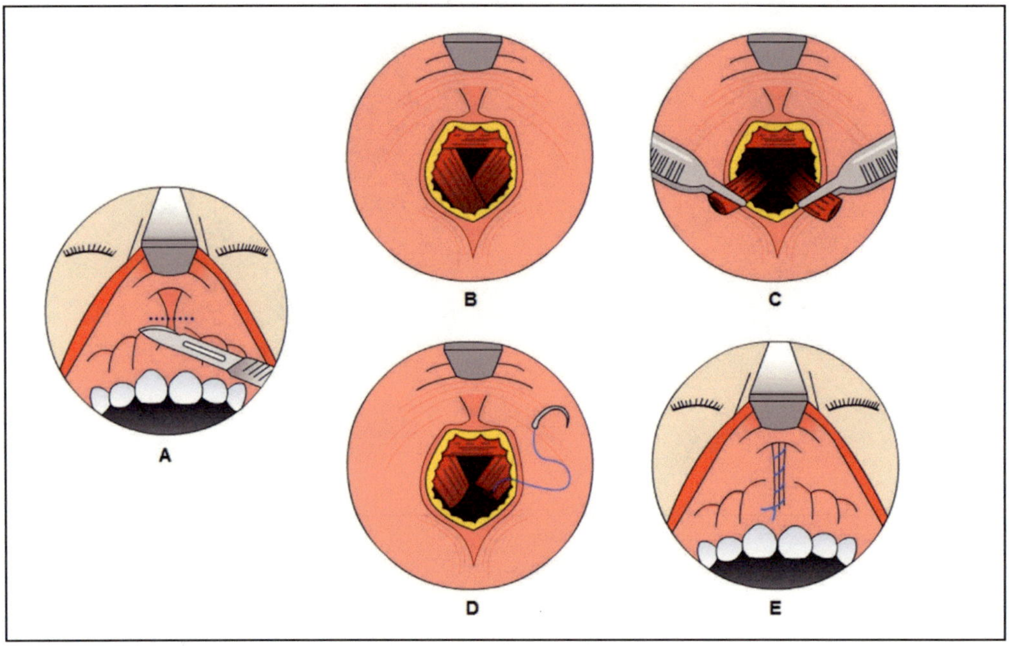

Figure 7. An artistic illustration of the transoral technique. a) Horizontal upper labial sulcus incision; b, c, d) Transposed and sutured to the contralateral transposed depressor septi nasi muscle; e) Close the horizontal incision vertically.

2.1. Transnasal technique

We infiltrate the membranous septum with 2% lidocaine with epinephrine 1:50,000, with a scalpel blade # 15 we make an incision of no more than 5 mm along the vestibular floor, the depressor septi nasi muscle is dissected and elevated with a dissecting Metzenbaum scissors from its position behind the columella, between the medial crura. Mahe and Camblin have noted that transaction of the depressor septi muscle may fail to produce lasting results because of reattachment of the muscle, that's why we prefer resect a 5-mm segment (Fig.8-9):

3. Nerve block of the depressor septi nasi muscle

For patients who don´t want a surgical treatment, we purpose the blocking of the depressor septi nasi with BNT-A for similar but temporary results, about 4 to 6 months. (Fig.10):

3.1. Trancutaneous technique

After patient selection, we mark the injection points at the base of the columella, two points at the medial crural footplate and one point between the two medial crura.

http://dx.doi.org/10.5772/62073

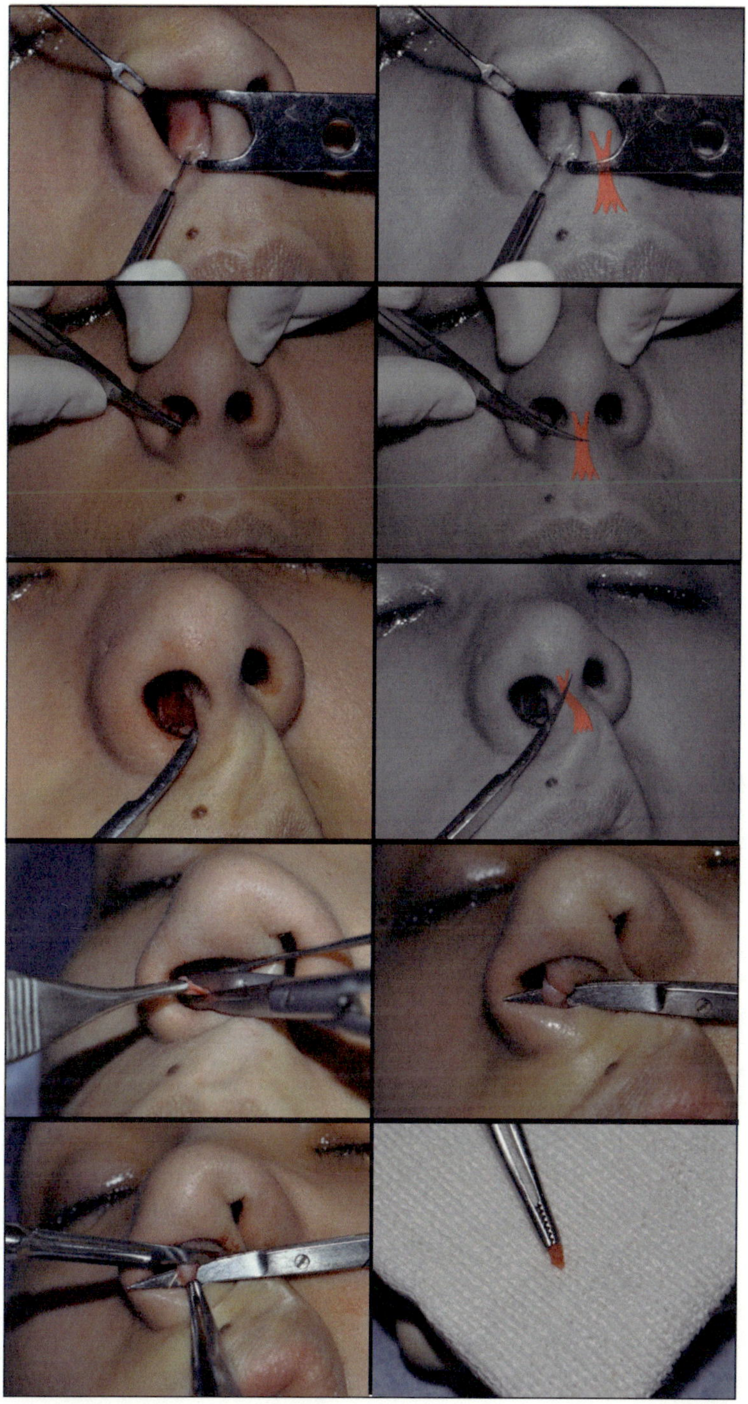

Figure 8. Transnasal technique.

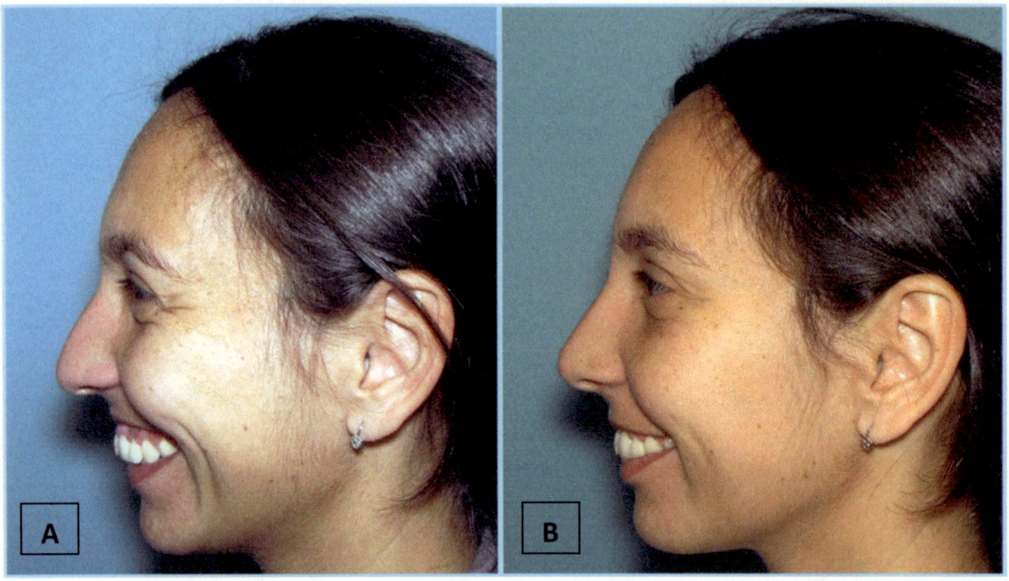

Figure 9. A) Preoperative patient with gingival smile, lowering of the nasal tip, upper lip shortening. and transverse crease in the mid-philtral area. B) Same patient in the pop period.

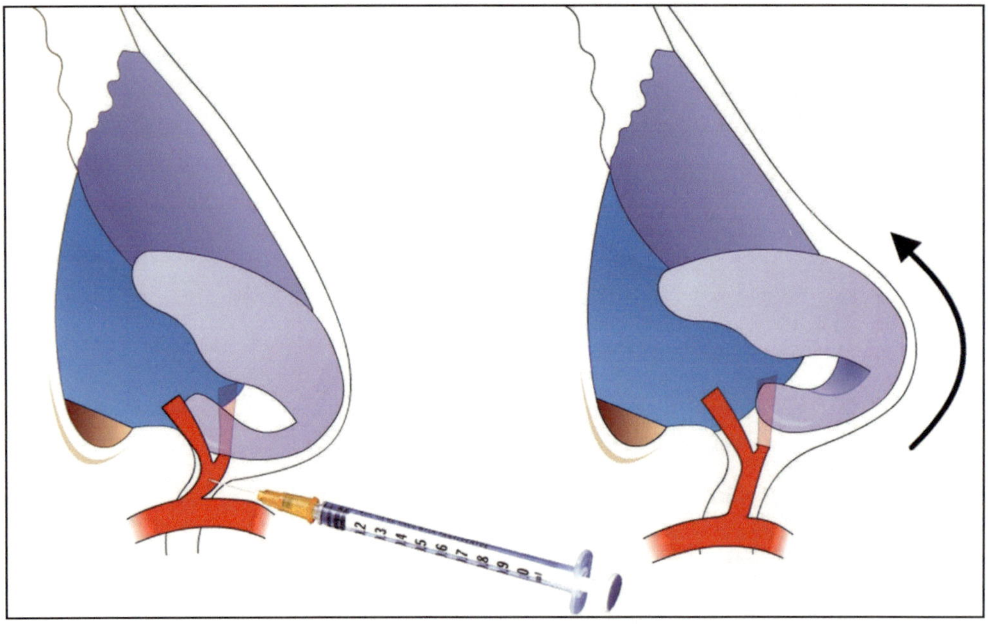

Figure 10. Nasal-labial angle blocking the m. depressor septi nasi with BNT-A: through the skin.

With a 1ml syringe and a 30G needle injecting 1 U of BNT-A at each point (Fig.11). After 1 week the results we get are relax the DSNM, enhancement of the nasolabial angle in static and dynamic positions, improvement the transverse crease in the mid-philtral area and prevent the dropping of the nasal tip during smile [8].

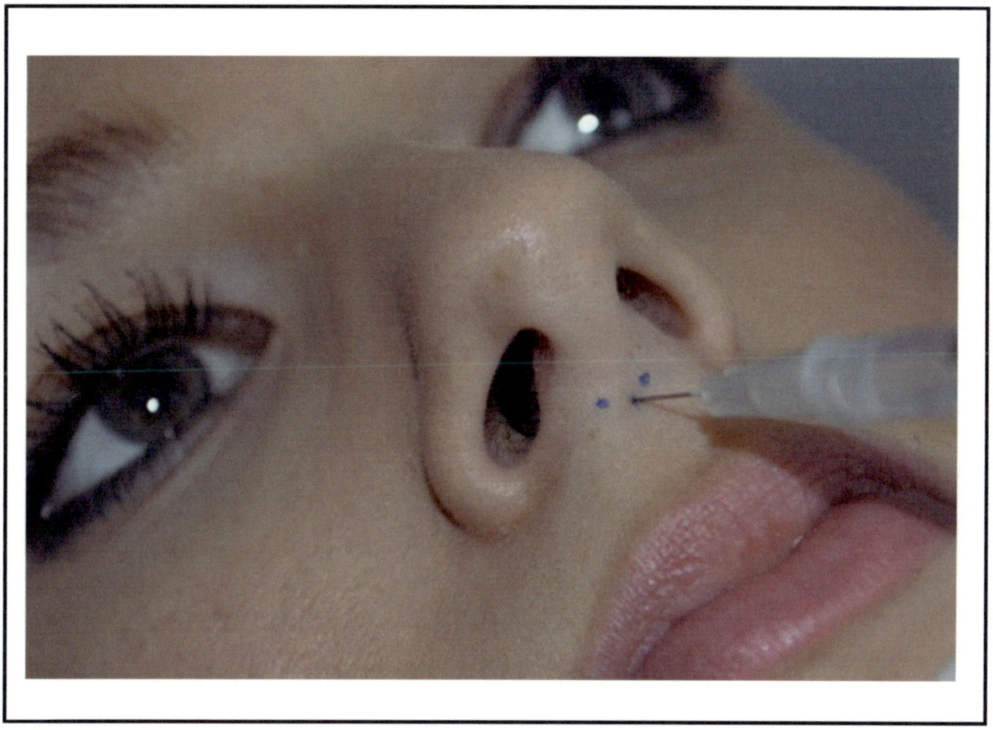

Figure 11. Nerve block of the DSNM technique.

4. Conclusion

An active depressor septi nasi muscle is responsible for descending the nasal tip, shortened upper lip, increased maxillary gingival show and transverse crease in the mid-philtral area. Those deformities can fixed with treatment minimally invasive with a permanent or temporary results

The authors of this chapter prefer the surgical treatment to get permanent results.

Acknowledgements

We would like to extend our grateful thanks to all those who helped make this chapter. Special thanks go to the following people:

To Jose Juri, M.D: Our master in Plastic and Reconstructive Surgery.

To Hector Moina, M.D for his willingness to review the chapter and his unfailing support.

To Gustavo Mouriño, M.D for his unconditional support.

To Alejandro Lucchelli, M.D for his high quality photography.

To Myrian Arenas, surgical scrub nurse, for her dedication.

Author details

Daniel G. Moina and Gabriel M. Moina*

*Address all correspondence to: dgmoina@hotmaill.com

Centro de Rinología y Cirugía plástica Dr Moina, Buenos Aires, Argentina

Conflict of interest
The authors have no conflicts of interest to disclose in relation this chapter.

References

[1] Rod J. Rohrich, Bang Hunyh, Arshad Muzaffar, William Adams and Jack Robinson.bImportance of the depressor septi nasi muscle in rhinoplasty: Anatomic study and clinical application. PlastReconstr Surg. 2000, January.

[2] J. Sainz Arregui, M. Elejalde, J. Regalado, F. Ezquerra and M. Berrazueta. Dynamic rhinoplasty for the plungings nasal tip: Functional unity of the inferior thirt of the nose.

[3] Cachay-Velásquez H. Rhinoplasty and facial expression.*Ann Plast Surg*. 1992;28:427–433.

[4] Abdoljalil Kalantar-Hormozi, Arash Beiraghi-Toosi. Smile analysis in rhinoplasty: A Randomized study for comparing resection and transposition of the depressor septi Nasi muscle. *Plast.Reconstr. Surg*. 133: 261, 2014.

[5] Rohrich RJ, Huynh B, Muzaffar AR, Adams WP Jr, Robinson JB Jr (2000) Importance of t he depressor septi nasi muscle in rhinoplasty: anatomic study and clinical application. Plast Reconstr. Surg 105:384–388

[6] Ebrahimi A, Nejadsarvari N, Motamedi MH, Rezaee M, Koushki ES (2012) Anatomic variations found on dissection of depresor septi nasi muscles in cadavers. Arch Facial Plast Surg 14:31–33.

[7] Jamil Ahmad, Rod Rohrich. Discussion: Smile Analysis in Rhinoplasty: A Randomized Study for Comparing Resection and Transposition of the Depressor Septi Nasi Muscle. Volume 133, Number 2. Discussion.

[8] Mauricio de Maio, Berthold Rzany: Botulinum Toxin in aesthetic medicine: Springer, 2007.

Chapter 8

Sutures or Resection of the Protruding End of Medial Crura

Daniel G. Moina and Gabriel M. Moina

Additional information is available at the end of the chapter

http://dx.doi.org/10.5772/62072

Abstract

The anatomic alterations of the columella may compromise aesthetically both the nasal base and its function.

This article describes how to diagnose compromised structures and how to solve them in a simple and minimally invasive way. In addition, we show how to anticipate the changes that we create according to the chosen technique in the nasal tip (the dynamic of the nasal tip).

Keywords: Medial crural, Nasal tip sutures, Footplates, Nasal tip, Nostril, Columella, Nostril test, Divergent alar cartilages, Asymmetrical footplates, Wide columella, Columella show, Rhinoplasty, Nasal defect, Nasal valves, Alar cartilage, Resection of the footplates, Deprojection of the nasal tip, Nasal base, Anatomical alterations of the columella, Narrow nostril

1. Introduction

1.1. Anatomy of the lateral alar crura

The nasal tip is supported by two arches composed of the lateral crura laterally, and the medial crura and the footplates medially. The medial crura function as pillars founded on the footplates.

The posterior 5–6 mm of the medial crura, which course laterally and often posteriorly, are called the footplates, and play a major role in the aesthetics of the nasal tip and therefore in rhinoplasty. The distance between the footplates ranges from 7.5 to 15 mm, the average being 11.4 mm.

Should the patient exhibit an overprojected tip, the result will be a divergent footplate (Fig. 1).

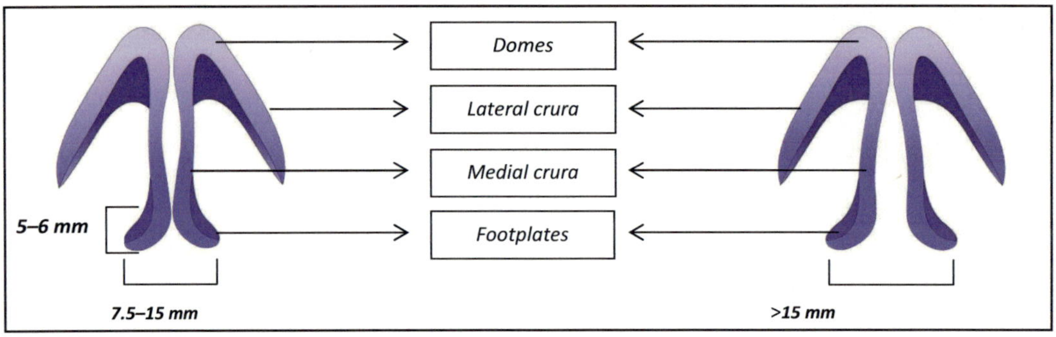

Figure 1. Anatomy of the lateral inferior cartilages with its portions, measures of its footplates (5–6 mm), normal distance between them (7.5–15 mm), and divergent lower lateral cartilages.

The columella is a relatively complex anatomical structure that is located in the nasal base between the nostrils. It is made of crura, muscle, skin, and soft tissue and does not only provide support to the nose but it is also an aesthetic component of great importance.

At the base of the columella the footplates protrude laterally giving amplitude to then adapt at the level of the medial crura. Deformities of the lower lateral cartilages lead to untoward aesthetics and functionality of the nostril and columella.

The ideal nostril possesses a teardrop shape with a long axis extending from the base to the apex. There is slight medial tilt of the long axis toward the midline (Fig. 2).

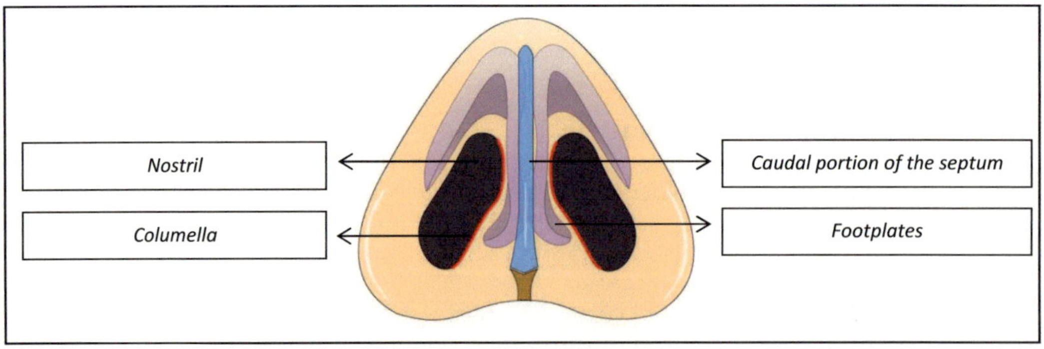

Figure 2. Nasal base which shows the columella, its cartilaginous structures, and the nostrils normal shape.

The columella shows a vast variety of deformities, anomalities, and variations that can result from genetic factors, trauma, altered growth, previous surgeries, or infections.The analysis of the deformity and its pathogenesis is of great importance as it will determine the surgical technique to follow.

In this article, we will focus on increasing the width of the columella as a result of one or both footplates being asymmetric in length, conformation (abnormally folded), and/or too separated and consequently protruding through the skin into the nasal vestibule. These entities may exist alone or in combination.

Anatomical alterations of the columella compromise the aesthetics of the nostrils and potentially its function, which is why the intimate relationship between nasal anatomy and physiology is crucial in rhinoplasty.

It is important to highlight that the ventilation can be affected especially when this alteration is combined with a narrow nostril, deviation or subluxation of the caudal portion of the nasal septum. A simple and effective method to evaluate this is the **Nostril Test** (test of columellar narrowing).

It consists of narrowing the lower third of the columella with bayonet forceps, this way we open the external nasal valve and ask the patient if this maneuver improves nasal ventilation (Fig. 3).

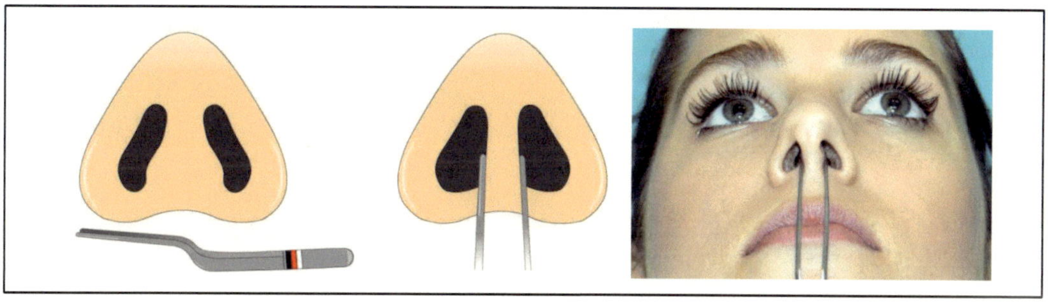

Figure 3. It can be observed how the base of the columella is narrowed by the bayonet forceps to evaluate if throughout this maneuver we generate any repercussion on the nasal ventilation (Nostril Test).

2. Etiopathogenesis

The causes that create an increase in the width of the columella can be divided into primary and secondary causes.

Primary causes: are those in which the alteration is in the lower lateral cartilages:

- Divergent alar cartilages associated with an excessive amount of soft tissue between the two intermediate pillars and footplates (Fig. 4a, b).
- Asymmetrical footplates in size and/or shape (retracted) (Figs. 5a, b).

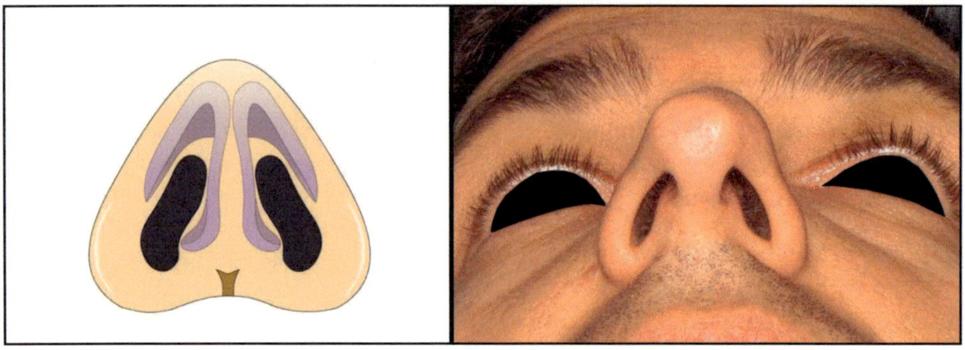

Figure 4. a, b) It can be observed how the columella widens symmetrically when both side pillars are divergent.

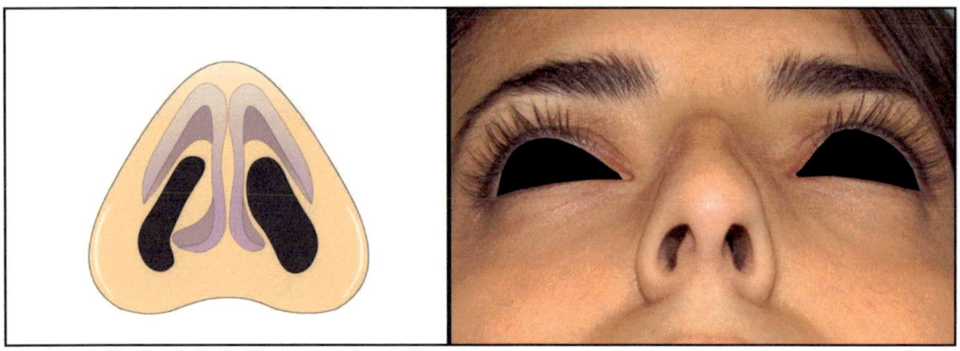

Figure 5. a, b) It can be observed how the columella widens asymmetrically at the expense of a longer and/or more bended lateral pillar.

Secondary causes: are those where there is an alteration of the medial pillars and footplates, either in shape and/or position triggered by adjacent structures (the caudal portion of the nasal septum and nasal spine).

- The deviation of the caudal portion of the nasal septum can displace the footplate of the alar cartilage and widen the columella (Fig. 6a, b).
- The deviation of the nasal spine can produce a deviated nasal septum and a displacement of the footplate of the alar cartilage and widen the columella (Fig. 7a, b).

http://dx.doi.org/10.5772/62072

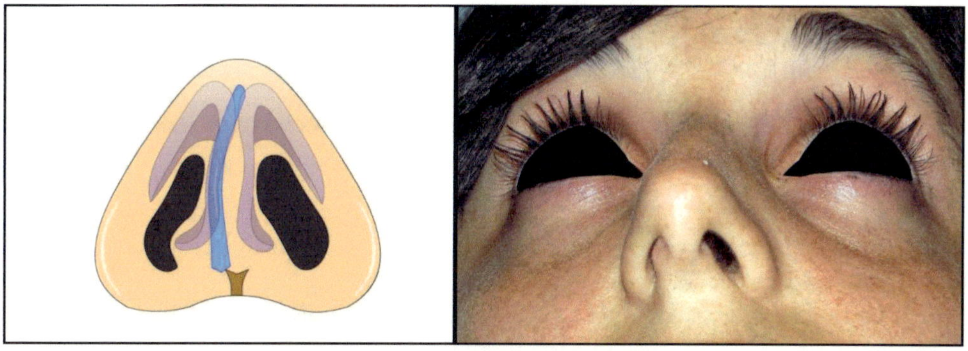

Figure 6. a, b) Deviation of the caudal portion of the nasal septum that produces a displacement of the footplate of the alar cartilage widening the columella.

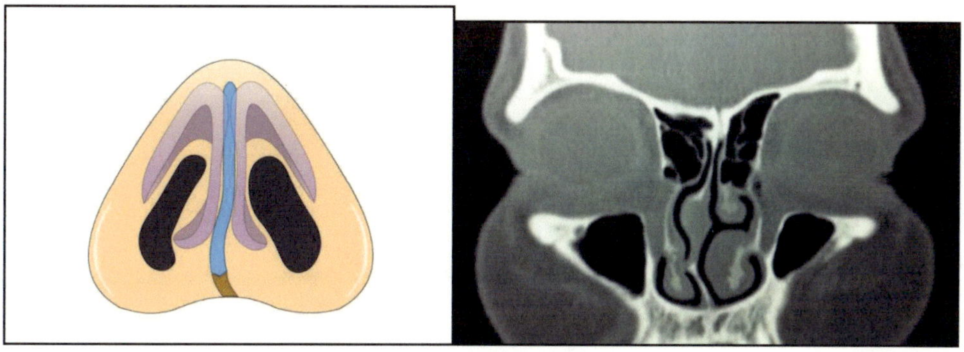

Figure 7. a, b) Deviation of the nasal spine that causes a slight deviation of the nasal septum, displacing the footplate of the alar cartilage, widening the columella.

In such cases, during surgery and with the individualization of the involved structures, the footplates of the alar cartilages tend to return to its usual position; however, the main pathology needs to be treated (septal deviation and/or nasal spine) and afterward the footplates of the alar cartilages have to be approximated by a stitch of transfixion.

NOTE: It is important that the described alteration (wide columella), regardless of etiology, can be solved with good results, the key to success is to make an accurate diagnosis, knowing the dynamics of the nasal tip, and choosing the appropriate surgical technique.

3. Surgical treatment of the wide columella through sutures

The suture between the feet of the lower lateral cartilages not only closes but stretches the base of the columella and improves the shape of the nostrils.

The lower lateral cartilages are the main suppliers of structural support of the nasal tip; therefore, any excess, shortfall, or alteration will directly affect not only the shape but also the position of the nasal tip.

It is important to note that the approximation of the footplates through sutures will not only produce the desired changes but will also trigger unwanted effects, if a thorough preoperative evaluation of the nose was not fully performed.

When suturing the footplates of the alar cartilages to approximate them, as mentioned above, we narrow the columella and improve the shape of the nostril; if there is a lot of soft tissue between them, a slight forward flow of the base of the columella (Fig. 8) will occur. Removing soft tissue between the footplates and the medial pillars before making the suture prevents such further protuberance on the columella when looking at the profile.

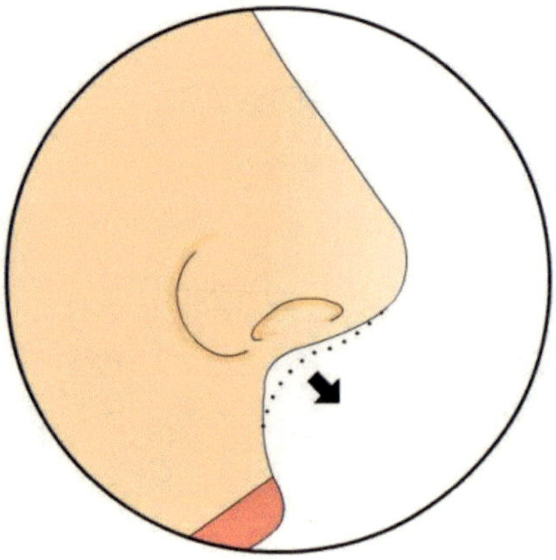

Figure 8. The dotted lines show the forward flow of the base of the columella after approximating the footplates of the alar cartilages by a stitch of transfixion.

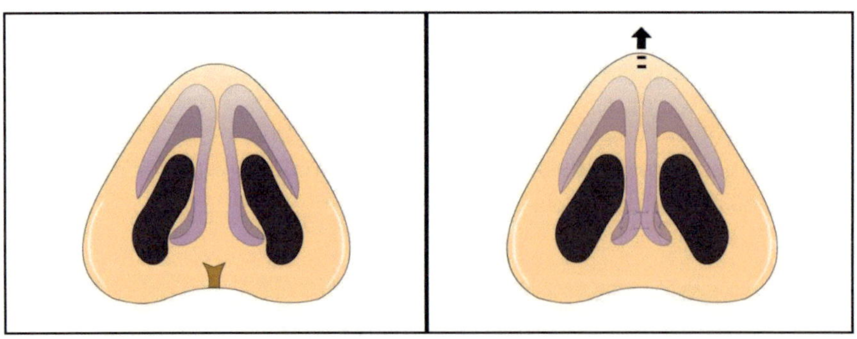

Figure 9. a, b) It is observed how the columella is refined and how the shape of the nostrils is improved through a transfixion stitch but also the nasal tip is slightly projected.

The approximation of the footplates will produce an increase of the tip projection, which means a positive effect if we have either a hypoprojected or normoprojected nose, but this is not a good suggestion if we are in presence of a hyperprojected nose (Fig. 9a,b), in which case you can resect a portion of the footplates and bring them closer with a stitch of transfixion.

3.1. Surgical technique

We infiltrate the membranous septum with 2% lidocaine with epinephrine 1:50,000; this way we produce analgesia, vasoconstriction, and a hydraulic detachment. Later on, with a scalpel blade # 11 we make an incision of no more than 3 mm above the membranous septum where the footplates protrude, and with curved Iris scissors we separate them from the mucous membrane and the soft tissue, then through a U stitch of transfixion with mononylon 4-0 we approximate them and close the 2 incisions made in the membranous septum with mononylon 6-0 (Fig. 10).

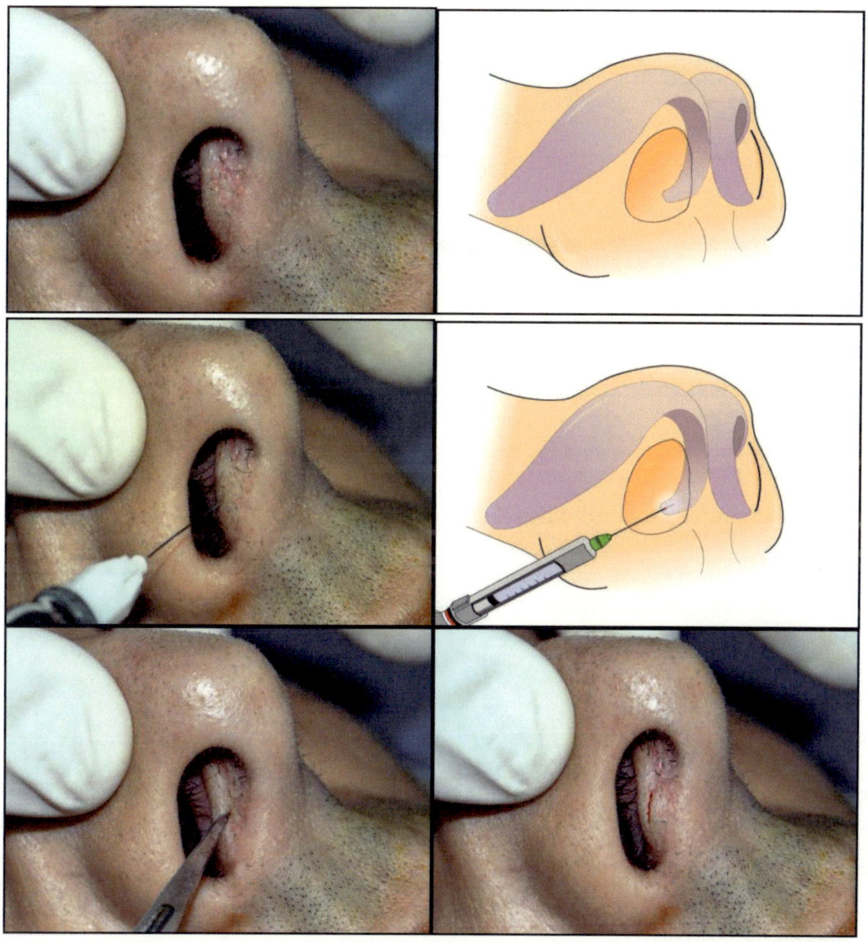

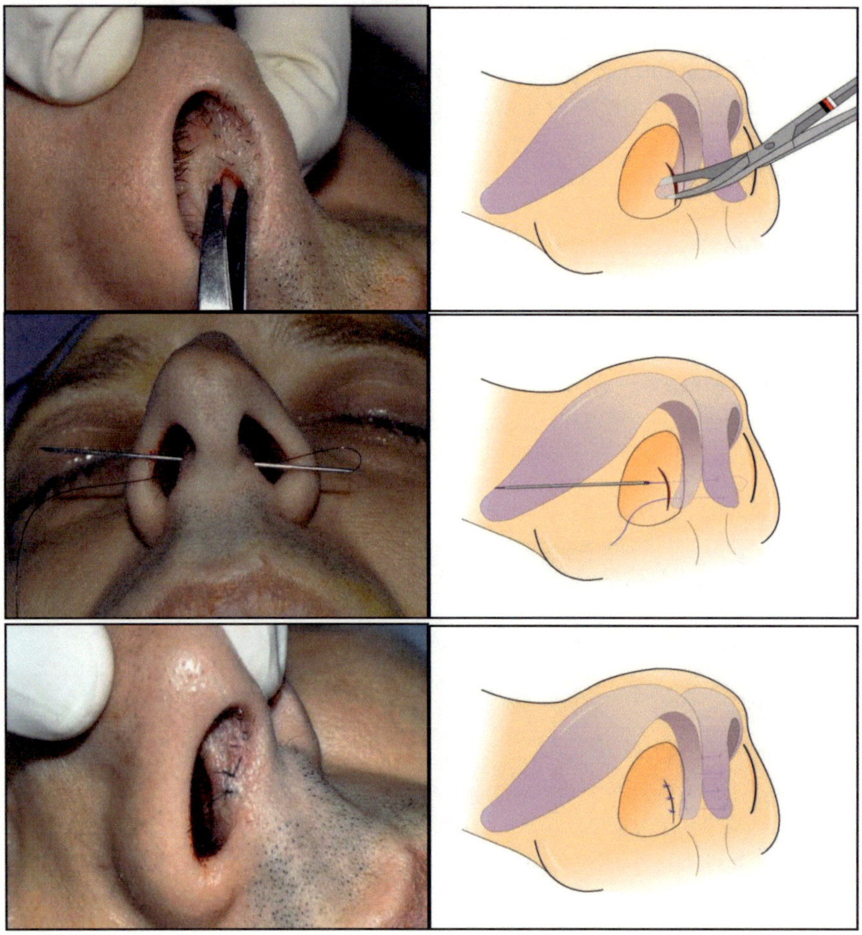

Figure 10. Surgical sequence where the approximation of the footplates is shown by a U stitch.

If necessary, we can add a second suture on the base to approximate the soft tissue (Fig. 11).

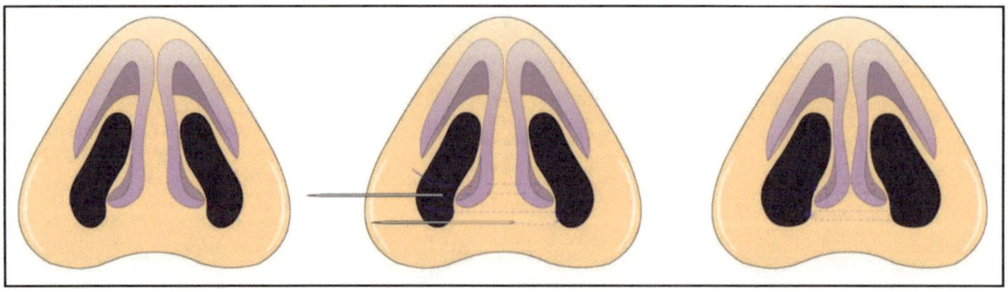

Figure 11. Surgical technique used for wide columella in cases where the footplates are divergent, symmetrical, and the nasal tip is hypoprojected or normoprojected, if necessary we add a second stitch of transfixion in the soft tissue to refine even more the columella.

http://dx.doi.org/10.5772/62072

4. Treatment of the wide columella by a resection of the footplates

The resection of the footplates of the alar cartilages is performed when these are asymmetric (a longer and/or more bent footplate) (Fig. 12a, b) or in case of divergent alar cartilages associated with a hyperprojected nasal tip (Fig. 13a, b), this way not only do we refine the columella and shape the nostril but we also accomplish a slight decline of the nasal tip.

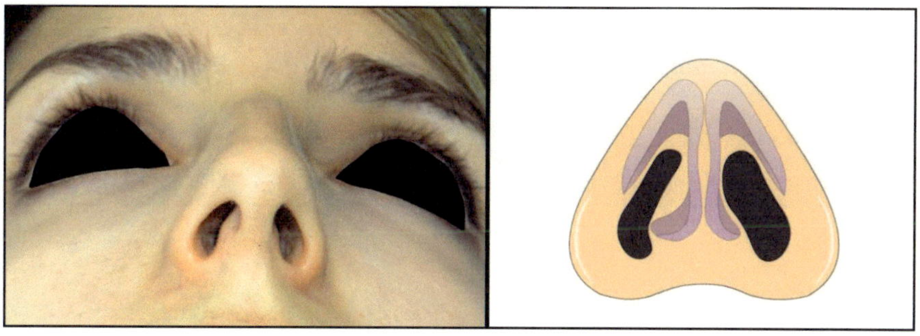

Figure 12. a, b) You can observe a wide columella; this is because the right footplate of the alar cartilage is more bent than usual.

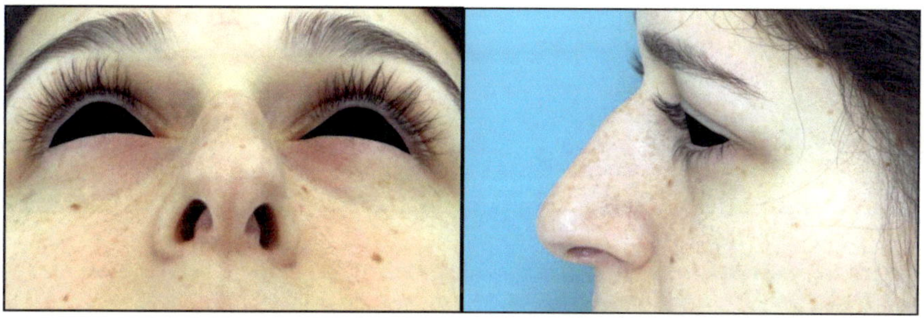

Figure 13. a, b) You can observe a widened columella in the nasal base as a result of divergent alar cartilages. The nasal tip is hyperprojected when looking at the profile, which is why the ideal surgical technique is the partial resection of the footplates and its posterior approximation by a U stitch transfixion.

4.1. Surgical technique

An infiltration with 2% lidocaine with epinephrine 1:50,000 is performed between the membranous septum and the footplates of the alar cartilages and between the divergent footplate and the soft tissue. We make a small 5 mm incision in the membranous septum at the level of the footplates with a scalpel blade # 11 and later on with Iris scissors we squeletize the divergent footplate of the alar cartilage (Fig. 14a, b). Note how in Fig. 15a, b, once the footplate is fully released it comes out easily. After that a portion of the footplate is resected with a sheet # 11 (Fig. 16a, b), then with a straight needle and a 4-0 mononylon the footplates are approximated by a U stitch transfixion; we make hemostasis control and close the incisions with mononylon 6-0 (Fig. 17a, b, c).

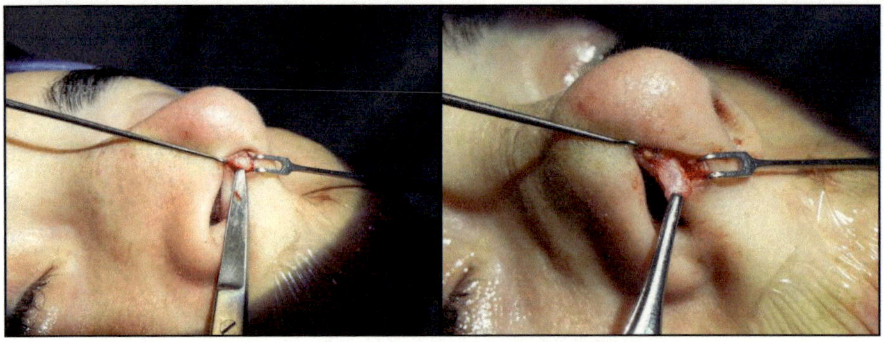

Figure 14. a, b) Dissection of the footplates of the divergent alar cartilages with Iris scissors.

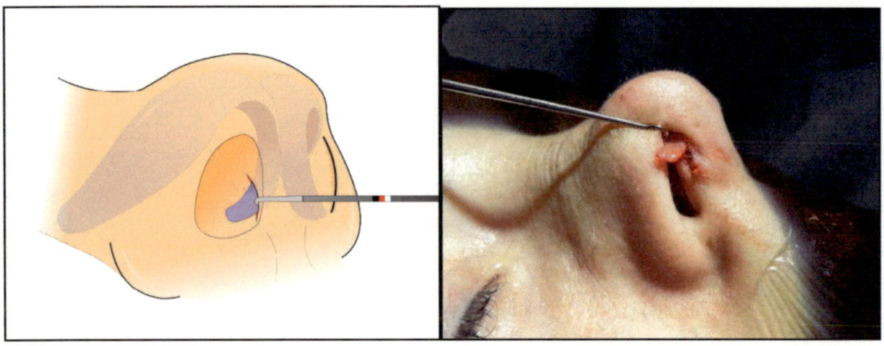

Figure 15. a, b) It is observed how once the footplates are fully released they are introduced into nostril.

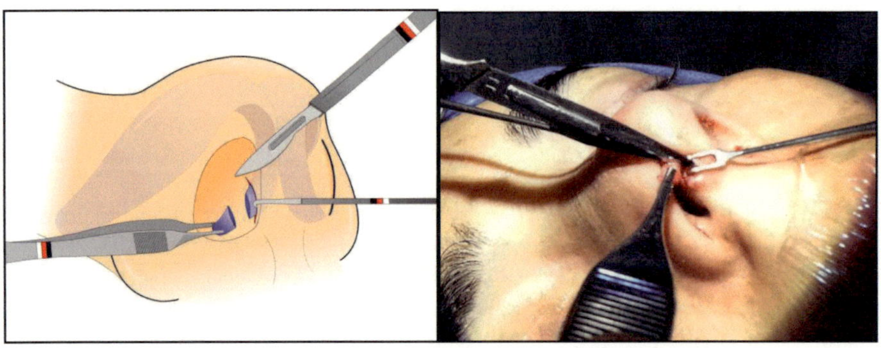

Figure 16. a, b) Resection of a portion of the footplates of the alar cartilage with a scalpel blade # 11.

http://dx.doi.org/10.5772/62072

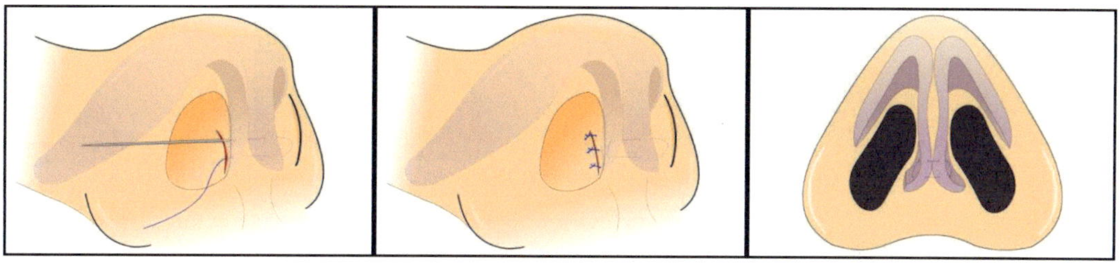

Figure 17. a, b, c) Making a U stitch of transfixion witch mononylon 4-0 and closing the membranous septum with mononylon 6-0.

In the following figures two surgical cases are shown:

Case 1: For a 25-year-old patient having a wide columella as a result of divergent footplates of the alar cartilages, it is decided to resect a portion of the footplates of the alar cartilages as the patient presents hyperprojected nose and in this way a minimal deprojection is also accomplished (Fig. 18).

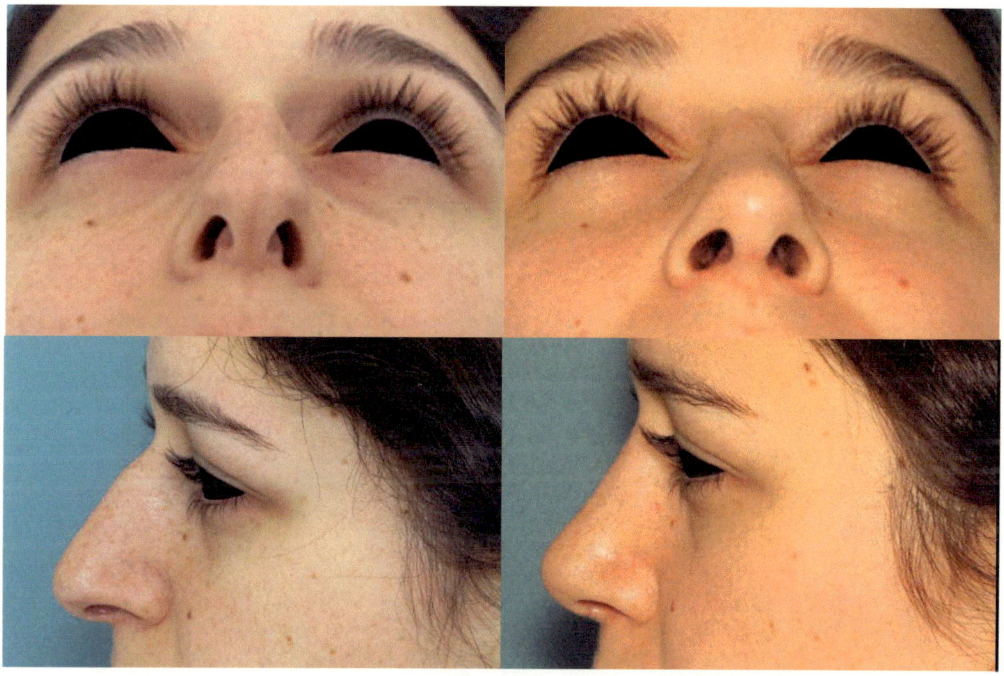

Figure 18. Pre- and postsurgical patient presenting divergent footplates.

Case 2: A 27-year-old patient shows at the examination of the nasal base a wide columella as a result of having a caudal septal deviation to the right and, consequently, this pushes the footplate ipsilaterally and protrudes into the nostril almost obliterating it completely (Fig. 19).

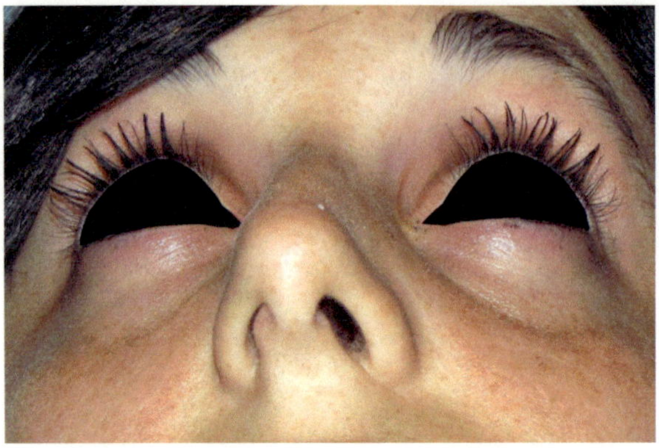

Figure 19. Dear Authors please add caption

The diagnosis is confirmed during surgery, where just by making a hemitransfixion incision on the membranous septum and releasing the nasal septum its caudal portion is deflected to the right (Fig. 20a, b). In this case, we center the nasal septum and join the footplates through point U of transfixion; in Fig. 21a, b, the pre- and postoperative photos are displayed.

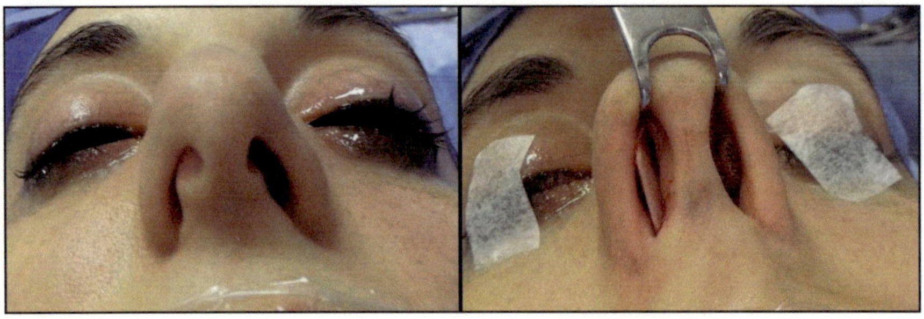

(a) (b)

Figure 20. Dear Authors please add caption

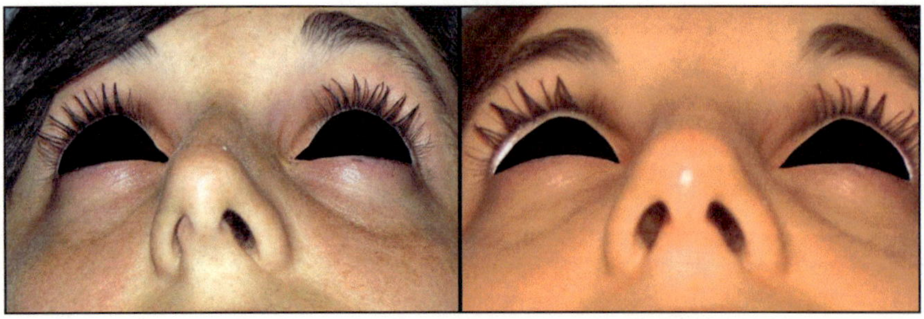

(a) (b)

Figure 21. Dear Authors please add caption

http://dx.doi.org/10.5772/62072

5. Conclusion

In this article, we try to show the reader that the nasal base is an aesthetic component that is as important as the dorsum or nasal tip, but surprisingly it does not get the attention it deserves and also that with detailed preoperative analysis and surgical or simple minimally invasive techniques we can achieve a symmetrical and harmonious nasal base.

Author details

Daniel G. Moina and Gabriel M. Moina*

*Address all correspondence to: dgmoina@hotmaill.com

Centro de Rinología y Cirugía plástica Dr. Moina, Buenos Aires, Argentina

Conflict of interest
The authors have no conflict of interest to disclose in relation to this article.

References

[1] Guyuron, B. Dynamics interplays during rhinoplasty. *Clin Plast Surg*. 1996;23: 223.

[2] Geiser P, Lee M, Roostaeian J, Unger J, and Rohrich R. Reshaping the medial nostril and columellar base: Five-step medial crural footplate approximation. *Plast Reconstr Surg*. 2013;132: 553.

[3] Cachay-Velásquez H, Languinge RE. Aesthetic treatment of the columella. *Ann Plast Surg*. 1989;22:370–379.

[4] Gruber, RP. Suture correction of nasal tip cartilage concavities. *Plast Reconstr Surg*. 1997;100: 1616.

[5] Guyron B. Footplates of the medial crura. *Plast Reconstr Surg*. 1998;101:1359–1363.

[6] Guyuron B. Dynamics in rhinoplasty. *Plast Reconstr Surg*. 2000;105:2257–2259.

[7] Baker, SR. Suture contouring of the nasal tip. *Arch Facial Plast Surg*. 2000;2: 34.

[8] Tardy, ME, Jr., Patt, BS, and Walter, MA. Transdomal suture refinement of the nasal tip: Long-term outcomes. *Facial Plast Surg*. 1993;9: 275.

[9] Guyuron, B, Uzzo, CD, and Scull, H. A practical classification of septonasal deviation and an effective guide to septal surgery. *Plast Reconstr Surg*. 1999;104: 2202.

[10] Gunter, JP, and Rohrich, RJ. Management of the deviated nose: The importance of septal reconstruction. *Clin Plast Surg*. 1988;15: 43.

Section 2

Non Surgical Techniques

Chapter 9

Medical Rhinoplasty – The Treatment of Mimical Patients

Alessio Redaelli

Additional information is available at the end of the chapter

http://dx.doi.org/10.5772/62071

Abstract

The plunging tip of the nose is a diffused cosmetically annoying problem. The medical rhinoplasty is a useful tool for the repair/reshaping of the plunging tip of the nose when the genesis is mimical. Botulinum toxin is used to repair this deformity. The anatomical details, the preparation of the materials, and the technique are discussed in this chapter with all the details that will permit the readers to understand and repeat the technique.

Keywords: Nasal profile, botulinum toxin A, mini-invasive rhinoplasty, nasal tip, muscles, nasal angles, depressor septi nasi, levator labii alaeque nasi, Dante's nose, plunging tip, hyper-projected nose, hypoprojected nose, aesthetics, beauty, aging

1. Introduction

The nose has always been one of the most important organs of our being. It characterizes indelibly our future habits from the very beginning of our life (such as the incredible example of salmons' olfactory imprinting at birth known as natal homing or natal philopatry: the homing process by which they travel for thousands of miles to breed in that particular stream where they were born) until death when we feel that particular smell of death [7,9].

In Chinese face reading, the nose is considered to be the money spot, especially during the ages of 41 to 50.

There is no place in the world where I go, where I am not asked to improve the appearance of the nose, no matter what the race, Asian or European, Afro-American or Japanese.

The nose determines the facial symmetry in a peremptory manner and represents our inner and outer bow. It is certainly one of the most exposed parts of our face to the attention of our partners, when we meet them for the first time. And this was especially true in the past centuries where also the figureheads (figureheads of ships) that adorned the bow of the ship put clearly in evidence the importance of nose (Fig.1), the bow of our thinking and being. It is therefore not strange that the technique published by me back in 2008 is today definitely one of the most widespread and known techniques of facial rejuvenation.

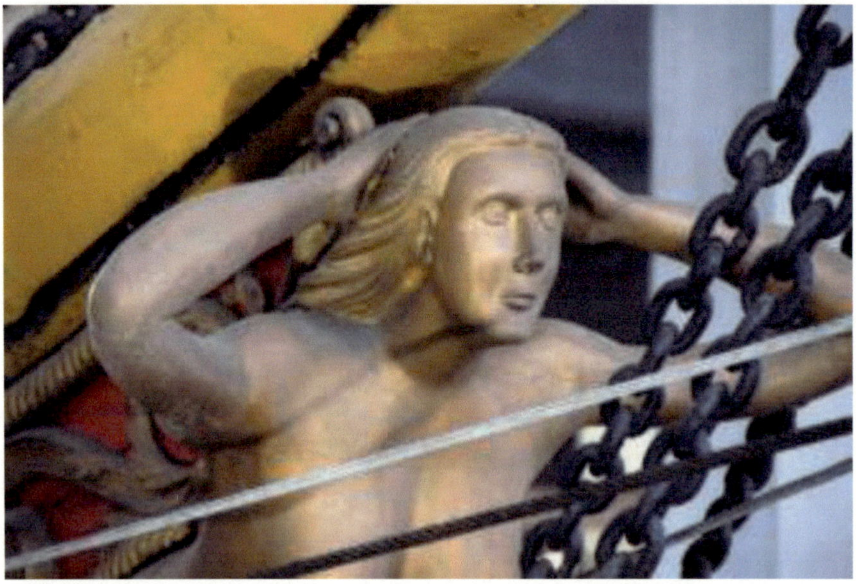

Figure 1. Figureheads of ships.

The facial aging is mainly due to three factors: the first is certainly the important reduction of volumes, the second the mimical movements with the arising of all the wrinkles on the face, and the third is due to the tone of the skin and subcutaneous tissue.

The exact understanding of the genesis of the defects we see all over the face provides the base for the treatments that we then adopt to repair these defects and the nose, of course, underlies these rules.

Knowing exactly when nasal defects became part of official medicine is impossible to date with precision. Egyptians 3000 years ago already knew about nasal surgery, also because of their important experience in embalming the dead. Even in China, because of the tradition of cutting the nose of adulterers, and many other types of criminals, there was a culture in the treatment of nasal defects. In the later period of the Middle Ages, several of these techniques became obsolete. But with the Renaissance there was a new impetus, particularly in Italy with the famous school of the Brancas, in Sicily and Gaspare Tagliacozzi (Bologna) [1]. The Branca and Gaspare Taglicozzi both are very famous for the so-called flap Italian (Fig. 2).

Probably, Jaques Joseph is the father of the modern surgical rhinoplasty, finding also a new method to reshape/repair the abnormally enlarged nasal wings (negroid nose) in black people (1904). But the first real medical rhinoplasty was most probably performed by the Belgian doctor Broeckaert [2] in 1901 (Fig. 3).

http://dx.doi.org/10.5772/62071

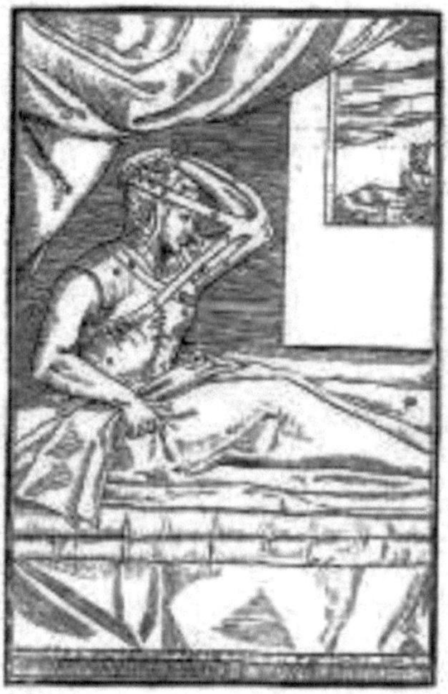

Figure 2. "Flap Italian."

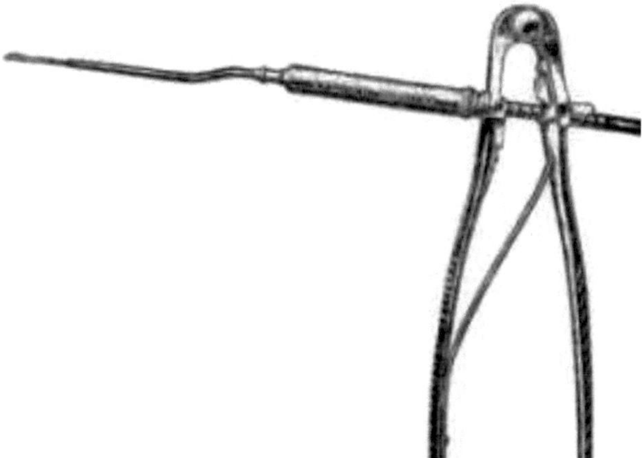

Figure 3. Broeckaert's syringe.

This doctor had invented a special syringe which was used to inject liquid paraffin (obtained also by pressure) in the soft tissues: here, I do not mention the side effects. We arrive finally to the present day with a huge improvement in all surgical techniques and with the advent of mini-invasive techniques and also of medical rhinoplasty, to be performed exclusively with medical techniques and, in detail, with the combination of botulinum toxin and fillers.

In my experience, over 80% of patients who arrive in our medical studies have major or minor nasal defects but only a small part of these patients, around 15–20%, agree to surgery. Others hesitate to meet the doctor for fear of undergoing an invasive and potentially dangerous procedure or because the defect, although sometimes clearly felt, is still very mild.

Finally, I want to mention that the nose is subject of the important phenomenon of aging just like all other areas of the face. It can get to present a drop of the tip up to 3–4 mm. In addition, a surgical nose perfectly corrected, and beautiful for a long time postsurgery, may after a few years begin to present some skeletonization that can be cured with a resorbable filler.

The main indications for medical rhinoplasty are:

- Aesthetical patients: mimical, volumetrical, and for deep bridge enhancement in Far East and African races.
- Surgical patients: the gold standard for correction is surgery, but they do not accept this solution, and so with medical rhinoplasty we can strike a good compromise.
- Postsurgical patients: to improve all those little postsurgical defects, once the object of a very difficult postsurgical reintervention.
- Functional patients: affected by atrophic rhinitis and atrophic generic problems to get a thicker mucosa.

In this chapter, we will focus mainly on patients with mimical deformity.

2. Anatomy

A quick reminder about anatomy [4,5,9,10] will be useful to readers. The skeleton is described in Fig. 4. Its main parts are the nasal bones, the alar triangular cartilages, the minor alar cartilages, and finally the Great (or major) alar cartilage. The vascularization starts from the lateral nasal vessels and columellar vessels arriving from the external carotid artery and the angular vessels arriving from the internal carotid artery and finally the dorsal nasal artery arriving from the frontal lobe. It is important during all the techniques described in this section to pay particular attention to these vessels that must not be injected.

In the nasal base, triangular, visible from the inferior projection, we can find in the middle the columella, while laterally the nasal wings are well-delineated by the lateral, intermediate, and medial crus of the greater alar cartilage.

The nasal muscles are visible in Fig. 5. The depressor septi nasi muscle and the levator labii alaeque nasi are most important for medical rhinoplasty. The depressor septi nasi muscle has a vector of contraction parallel to the columella and pushes the nasal tip toward the maxillar bone. The levator labii alaeque nasi (elevator of the lip and nasal wings), instead, elevates the nasal wings, contemporaneous with the lip. So we can describe a real rotational movement that characterizes some individuals (Fig. 6).

http://dx.doi.org/10.5772/62071

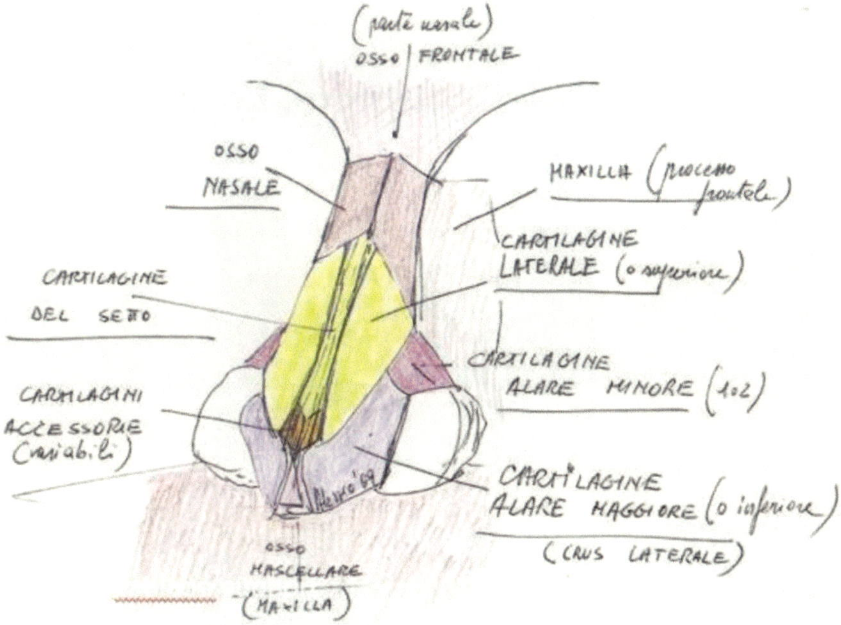

Figure 4. Bones and cartilages of the nose.

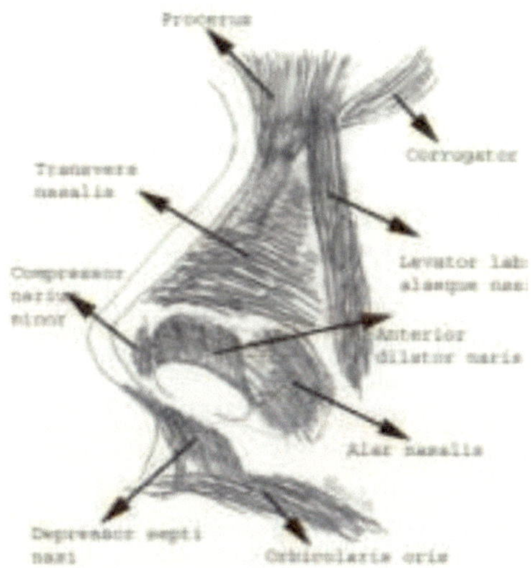

Figure 5. Bones and cartilages of the nose.

The superficial layer is characterized deeply by a superficial fascia that covers all the nasal muscles, extension of the facial SMAS. The subcutaneous layer and epidermis are characterized

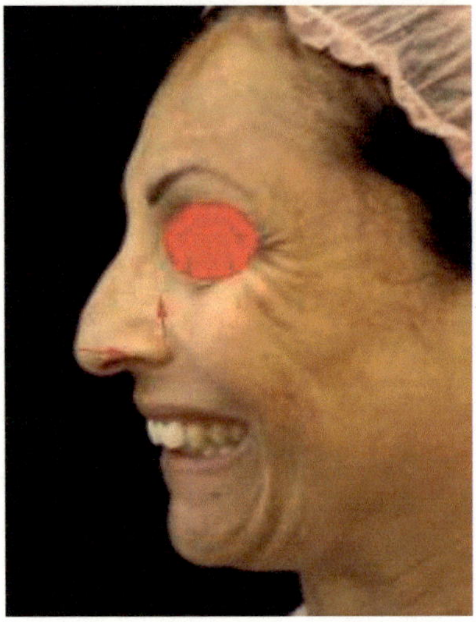

Figure 6. Nasal motion arrows.

by a thick and less adherent skin at the root of the nose, a very thin and more adherent skin in the middle, and finally a thicker and also adherent skin that covers the tip of the nose.

3. Aesthetical study

The aesthetical study is based as always on strict rules. All the measures of the face have been described many centuries ago by Italian scientists like Leonardo da Vinci and must be exactly known by every doctor who wants to use this technique.

The main nasal points of interest are described in Fig. 7. The nasal area is from the Glabella to the Nasal spin through Nasion, Rhinion, and Nasal tip.

In the same figure, it is possible to study the main nasal angles: nasofrontal angle, from 115° to 135°; dorsal angle, normally straight or slightly lower; nasolabial angle, from 90° to 110°.

In the perfect aesthetical indication, the nasofrontal and nasolabial angles are slightly reduced, while the dorsal angle is a bit increased (see Fig. 7).

Table 1 lists the main aesthetical indications.

The nose is generally connected to all other areas of the face, particularly the malar area, the lips, and the chin [10]. In particular, Angle's classes are of great importance. I will not dwell too much on their description since this can be studied accurately in many specific texts. I would only emphasize on the importance of Ricketts' e-line, which connects the tip of the nose with the Pogonion. It will always be of great importance to control the real projection of the chin and areas around the nose. It will be of evidence how even a rather long and hyperpro-

http://dx.doi.org/10.5772/62071

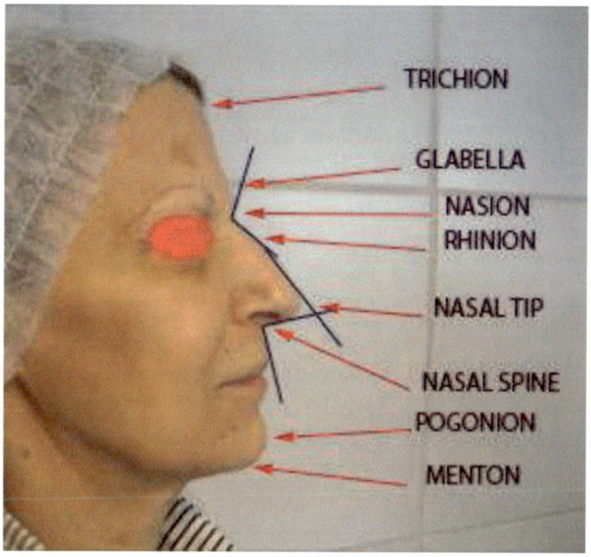

Figure 7. Nasal points of interest.

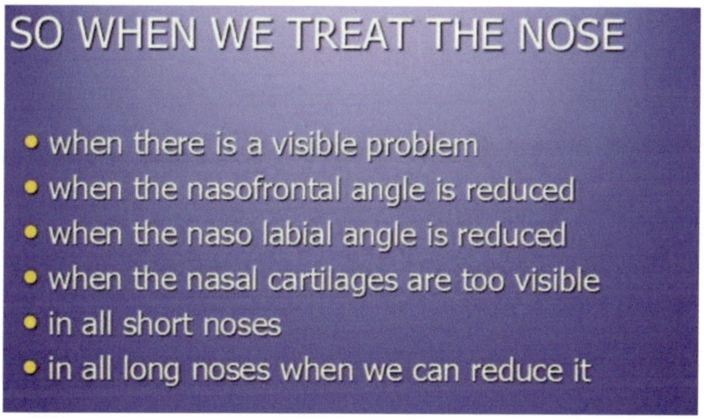

Table 1. Aesthetical indications.

jected nose may be such that, in some cases, for an opposite hypoprojection of the zygomatic-malar and mental areas, for example, in a second skeletal class. (Fig. 8)

4. Treatment of mimical patients

In a wide number of studies, it is confirmed that about 60% of patients with the typical plunging tip of the nose present a really mimical genesis for the hyperactivity of the depressor septi nasi (depressor of the nasal tip) or the levator labii alaeque nasi (elevator of the lip and nasal wing).

The treatment of these patients is based on the use of Botulinum toxin A.

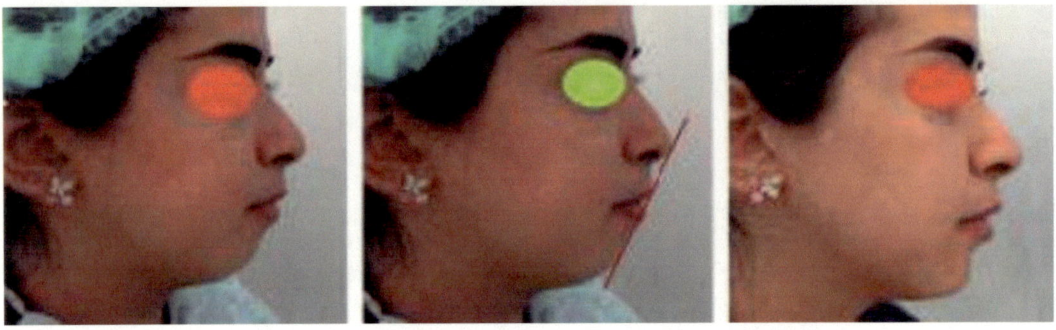

Figure 8. The importance of the chin. An interesting case of a Middle Eastern patient, 2′ skeletal class, who was treated with a filler on the chin, before and after treatment. It is immediately possible to see how many changes occur as well as the projection of the nose, and overall changes on the whole face.

Botulinum Toxin A (BTxA) is a neurotoxin approved in many countries and also in Europe. Its "On-Label" use is in the glabellar region. Other uses and also the treatment of mimical patients with the plunging nasal tip, include an "Off-Label" indication.

While for an "On-Label" treatment, the informed consent could even be oral (although I always ask the patient to sign up in writing anyway), in all "Off-Label" indications I remind all readers that the informed consent must necessarily be in writing.

All classical contraindications of BTxA must be completely investigated and as always in medicine a complete anamnesis must be done. We cannot treat patients with myasthenia and myastenic form syndromes (Lambert Eaton) and patients who are allergic to components of the product.

Patients requiring a fine control of the movements of the upper lip, and peri-oral area, like the players of musical instrument or singers, are a strict contraindication.

4.1. Materials approved in Europe

The materials approved in Europe (Fig. 9) are:

- **Vistabel/Vistabex/Cosmetic Botox**: Derived from **Botox**, Allergan, Irvin California. It can be stored in the refrigerator between 2° and 8° and it is in vials of 50 or 100 U.
- **Azzalure**: Distributed in Europe by Galderma, directly derives from **Dysport**, Ipsen. It is moderately stronger than Botox; it must be stored in a refrigerator between 2° and 8° and is available in vials of 125 U.
- **Bocouture**: Distributed in Europe by Merz, directly derives from Xeomin. In Europe, it is available in vials of 50 U. It can be stored at room temperature.

The different preparations are not interchangeable and the specific units are diverse, just like their action in the tissues.

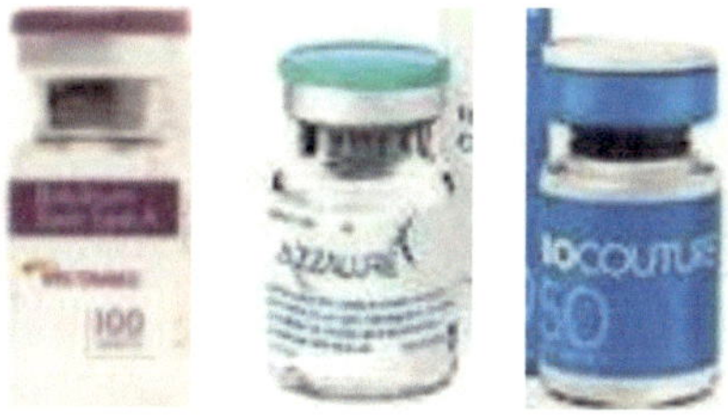

Figure 9. Materials approved in Europe.

4.2. Preparation of materials

All the materials are in a dry-vacuum vial and must be prepared just prior to the treatment. For the dilution, physiological solution is normally used [3,8].

Vistabel 50 U is diluted with 1.25 ml (1 U in 0.025 and 4 U in 0.1 ml). Azzalure 125 U is diluted with 0.63 ml (5 U in 0.025 and 20 U in 0.1 ml). Bocouture 50 U is diluted with 1.25 U (1 U in 0.025 and 4 U in 0.1 ml)

In particular conditions (for particularly fine areas as for example the mouth, to treat very thin muscles, etc.), it is possible to dilute less to obtain a very concentrated material. If we dilute less or more, the U contained in the final solution will be accordingly different.

Why do I often dilute less? What is the philosophy behind this concept? If the readers check the specifications in the leaflet inside the vials, they will find that some side effects such as headache, ocular disorders such as blepharo-ptosis, and eyelid edema are likely to occur (between 1/10 and 1/100). I believe that these side effects can be due to the excessive dilution. This can lead to an excessive spread of the toxin in anatomical regions that are too close not to be affected by its effect (such as the upper eyelid). This can happen especially in some patients with particular kind of atonic tissues. Prudence in aesthetic medicine is one of the most important issues to follow.

Finally, I want to highlight the syringe I use normally, a 0.5 ml syringe for diabetes or, better, a 0.3 ml syringe for diabetes with inserted needle 30 G x 8 mm. The demi-type syringe is perfect (Fig. 10).

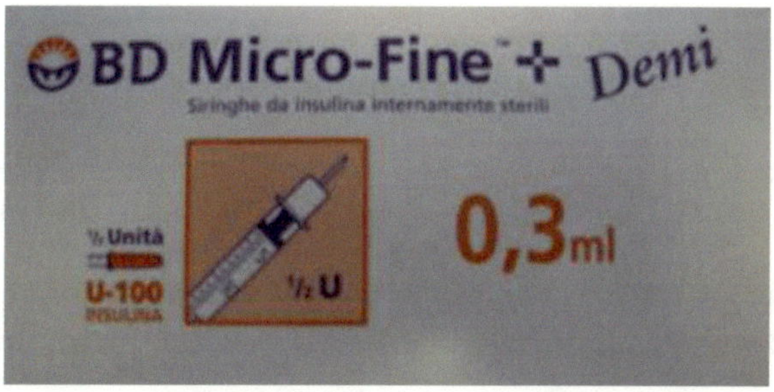

Figure 10. A demi-type 0.3 syringe.

4.3. Study of patients

Before the treatment of mimical patients, it is mandatory to completely study their movement, to exactly understand if there is an indication to the treatment and which muscles must be injected. For this reason, we have a moment that is so important to understand the movements: the first 2 or 3 minutes of the visit, when we give our hand to the patient and she/he is completely natural, and moves without being conscious of being observed.

In these first moments of the visit we have the opportunity to see the nasal tip that is much depressed in mimical patients, and especially if we have to see the rotational movement, we speak few lines before.

In the majority of patients, we can see the typical movement of the depressor septi nasi: the tip of the nose is pushed down toward the maxillar bone (Fig. 11 b). In such patients, it is possible to see also the contemporary movement of the levator labii alaeque nasi as the nasal wings can arise. At the same time, the nasolabial angle tends to reduce, much lower than 90°.

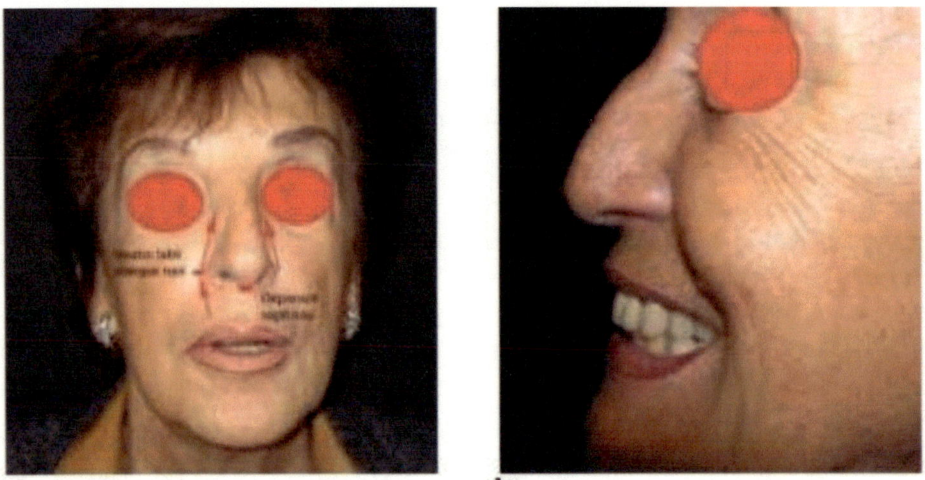

a b

Figure 11. A mimical patient is studied before the treatment in frontal projection (a) and in profile (b)

4.4. Treatment of the "Depressor septinasi" muscle

The depressor septi nasi muscle, as described earlier, is inserted on the maxillar bone at the nasal spine. Its fibers rise toward the nasal tip through the columella [8,9].

This treatment is based on the injection of fibers or in the colummella or at the nasal spine. I normally use a 0.5 ml syringe for diabetes. I inject 4 U Vistabel/Bocouture or 10U Azzalure.

The left hand opens the side of the columella to be injected, making also a light rotation of the nasal base.

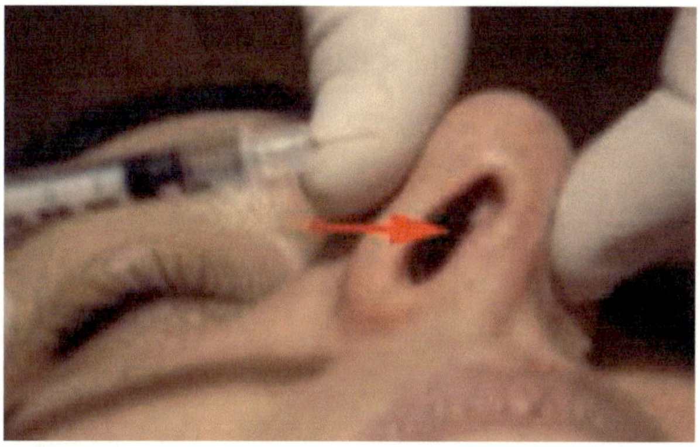

Figure 12. Injection of the columella.

The other hand holds the syringe and injects perpendicularly to the columella axis (Fig. 12). If we inject the muscle along the columella, the risk of affecting nearby muscles is usually nil.

It is possible also to inject the muscle at the nasal spine (Fig. 13). In this case, it is possible also that a very small quantity of toxin can spread in some fibers of the nearby muscles, especially the Buxinator muscle that makes the deep muscular layer around the lips. This is the reason why some patients come back for a retouch 15 days later, reporting sometimes that they feel a bite in their cheeks: the buxinator muscle, for some days, partially loses its precision in keeping food under the teeth. It disappears by time and a useful advice for patients regarding this possible side effect is to pay attention to chewing.

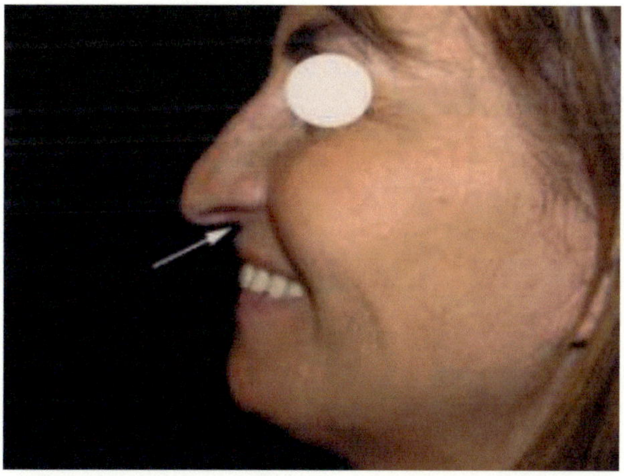

Figure 13. The nasal spine.

4.5. Treatment of the "elevator of the lip and nasal wing" muscle

In Fig. 13, it is possible to see the important elevation of the nasal wing up and laterally, clearly visible in the profile projection. This is very important especially in black and Far East races, where the widening of the nasal base while smiling is very typical.

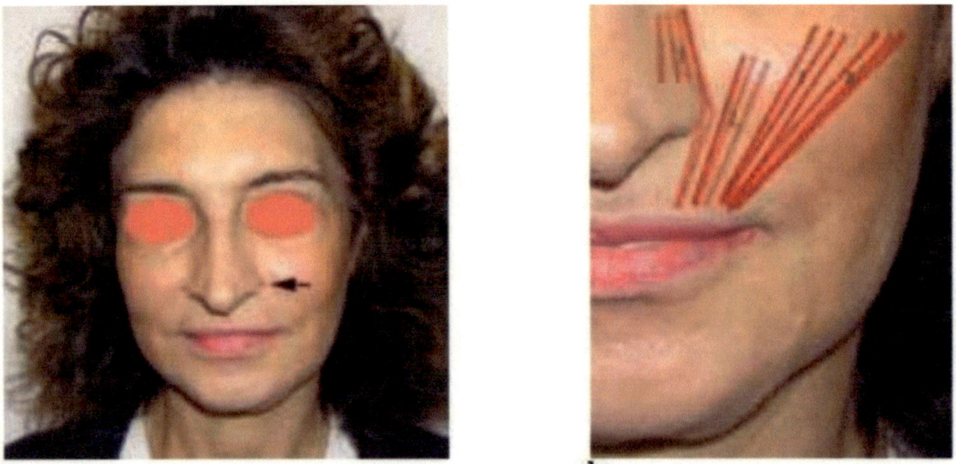

a b

Figure 14. Points of injection of "levator labii alaeque nasi" muscle (a). In (b) it is possible to see the position of the elevator muscles of the upper lip: 1 – levator labii alaeque nasi, 2 – elevator of the lip, 3 – zygomaticus minor, 4 – zygomaticus major.

In Fig. 14a and b, it is possible to see the injection points and the elevator muscles of the upper lip.

Normally, I inject at the elevator of the lip and nasal wing at their half, just laterally to the nasal wings, as visible in Fig. 14a. It is important to remain medially, since just laterally to this muscle we find the elevator of the lip [8,9].

As has been said many times, it is of great importance to study the patients. So, if we have a concomitant gummy smile, the risk of injections will be very low. Otherwise, if we do not want definitely a lip lowering, we will remain totally in the "elevator of the lip and nasal wing" [8].

So if we have a concomitant gummy smile, we want a greater spread of the toxin and I dilute with the normal dilution (1.25 ml for Vistabel/Bocouture and 0.63 for Azzalure) or even more.

If, instead, I want to avoid any spreading in nearby muscles I will dilute the material with a lesser quantity of physiological water (1 ml for Vistabel/Bocouture and 0.5 for Azzalure).

There is no real rule about the number of Units to use, but if we want to remain prudent I suggest the readers not inject more than 4 U Vistabel/Botox/Bocouture/Xeomin or 5 U Azzalure/Dysport.

Example 1:

In the case of a 63-year-old patient who comes to me for the treatment of BTxA for facial wrinkles, in the study prior to treatment it is possible to clearly see the depression of the nasal tip by muscular genesis.

She has a good indication for the treatment of nasal depression muscles.

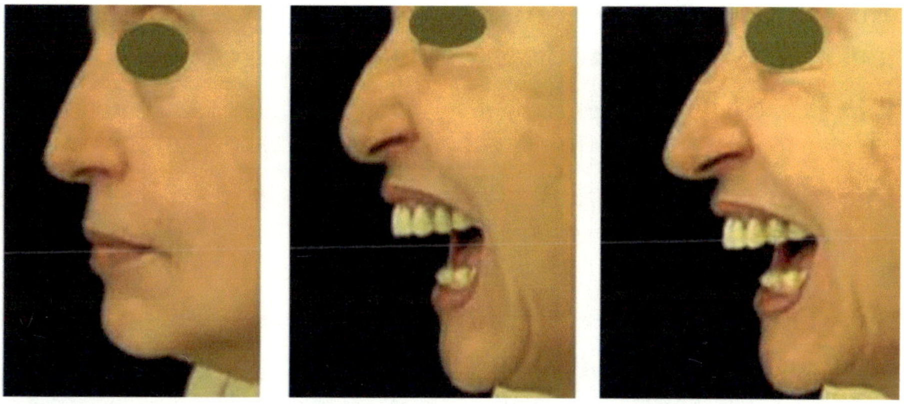

Figure 15. The patient is studied before in basic position (a), during movement (b), and after 15 days (c).

The patient was treated only in the columellar injection point with 2 U Vistabex per side. I used a 0.5 ml syringe and the dilution used was with 1.25 ml.

I probably made a mistake not to treat also the levator labii alaeque nasi, since the movement was very important and especially after 15 days it was more visible, compared with the image of the movement before the procedure.

Author details

Alessio Redaelli*

Address all correspondence to: mail@docredaelli.com

Visconti di Modrone Medical Center, Milan, Italy

References

[1] Tagliacozzi G. De curtorum chirurgia per insitionem. Venezia; 1597.

[2] Broeckaert J. Prothèse nasale au moyen d'injections de paraffine. Gand; 1901.

[3] Redaelli A. Botulinum toxin dilution: our technique. *J Cosm Laser Ther* 2003; 5: 218–219.

[4] Dayan SH, Kempiners JJ. Treatment of the lower third of the nose and dynamic nasal tip ptosis with Botox. *Plast Reconstr Surg* 2005; 115(6): 1784–1785.

[5] Rohrich RJ, Huynh B, Muzaffar AR, et al. Importance of the depressor septi nasi muscle in rhinoplasty: anatomic study and clinical application. *Plast Reconstr Surg* 2000; 105(1): 376–383; discussion 84–88.

[6] Redaelli A. *The Aesthetic Medicine*. Firenze: See-Editrice; 2009.

[7] Redaelli A. Medical rhinoplasty with hyaluronic acid and botulinum toxin A: a very simple and quite effective technique. *J Cosm Dermatol* 2008; 7, 210–220.

[8] Redaelli A. *The Botulinum Toxin A in Aesthetic Medicine, for the Treatment of Hyperhidrosis and in Odontostomatology: Basic Principles and Clinical Practice*. 2nd ed. Firenze: OEO; 2012.

[9] Redaelli A., Braccini F. *The Medical Rhinoplasty: Basic Principles and Clinical Practice.* Firenze: OEO; 2010.

[10] Redaelli A, Braccini F. *Facial Aging: Medical, Surgical and Odontostomatological Solutions*. Firenze: OEO; 2011.

Chapter 10

Botulinum Toxin in the Nasal Area

Diego Schavelzon, Guillermo Blugerman, Gabriel Wexler and Lorena Martinez

Additional information is available at the end of the chapter

http://dx.doi.org/10.5772/62070

Abstract

Introduction: Botulinum toxin type A for aesthetic purposes has been used since 1987, proving to be one of the most popular procedures in aesthetics due to its effectiveness in softening dynamic wrinkles.

Nasoglabellar lines or bunny lines:They are the result of the contraction of the nasal transversus. They can be primary or secondary, the latter as a result of muscle blockade in glabellar region, generating a compensatory contraction.

Specific application

Nasal tip ptosis: As people age the nasal tip tends to fall due to gravity forces and due to the kinetic action of the depressor of the septum muscle. The application of Botox in this area will only have positive results if the ptosis is of muscular cause.

Nasal flutter: Physical or emotional stress causes the involuntary contraction of the anterior and posterior dilator naris. Also the injection in these muscles produces the stretching of nostrils of very wide noses, when these muscles are active (they can move the ala).

Hyperhidrosis of nasal dorsum: The precise diagnosis of the areas is done through the Minor test (iodinated alcohol and starch). The injection is done in the dermis until the skin turns white, 1– 2 UI per injection, separating them by 1cm.

Multiple eccrine hidrocystomas: This papula-cystic lesion, described by Andrew Ross Robinson, has a transparent dome through which a blue color is seen, usually confused with blackhead. They originate in sweat ducts and come out associated with hyperhidrosis.

Keywords: BOTOX nasal applications, Botulinum toxin, bunny lines, dynamic wrinkles, gingival smile, nasal anatomy, nasal cosmetic procedures, nasal dermatology, nasal dynamics, nasal flutter, nasal hyperhidrosis, nasal muscles, nasal proportions, nasal tip ptosis, nose aesthetics, multiple eccrine hidrocystomas, minimal invasive procedures, muscle blockade, wide nose

1. Introduction

Since 1987, Botulinum toxin type A has been used to enhance the aesthetic appearance of the upper third of the face (Fig. 1). The main effect is softening of dynamic wrinkles by diminishing mimic muscles contraction. Nowadays, the cosmetic use of Botulinum toxin is no longer limited to this area and has extended to the inferior third of face, neck, and the medial facial area and to the nose, which is the main subject of this book.

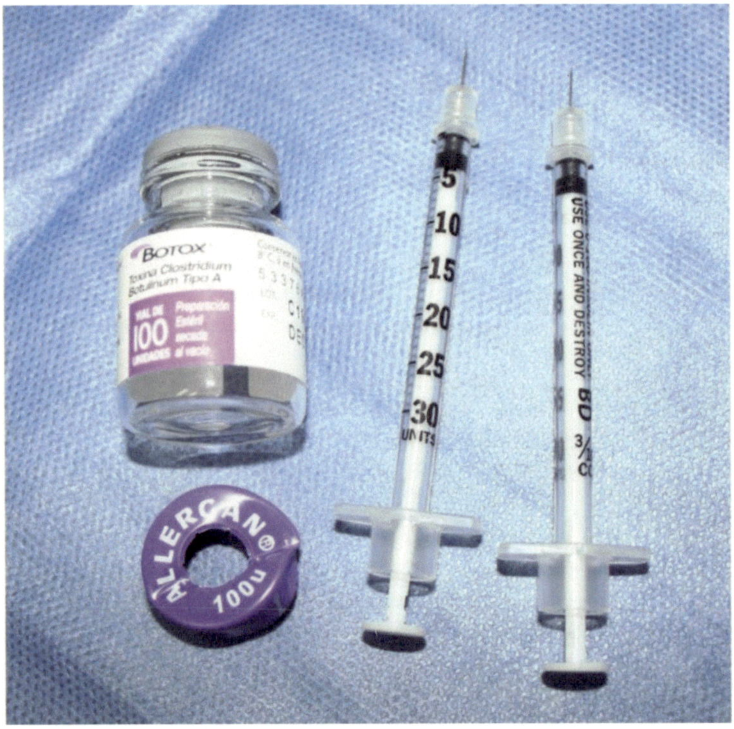

Figure 1. Commercial presentation of Botox®. Syringes used for application.

Botulinum toxin type A's popularity has increased in the past years, proving to be the most popular aesthetic procedure in the world, according to international scientific societies, mainly due to its safety and predictable results. We have large experience in the use of Botulinum toxin in the nose and other facial areas. In this chapter, we will share our experience with Botulinum toxin type A in nasal muscles.

1.1. Nasal muscles

According to Latourneau and Daniel [1], the superficial musculoaponeurotic system (SMAS) that covers the nasal dorsum and ala is composed by eight muscles that share common fascias with neighboring areas such as lids, cheeks, lips, and forehead.

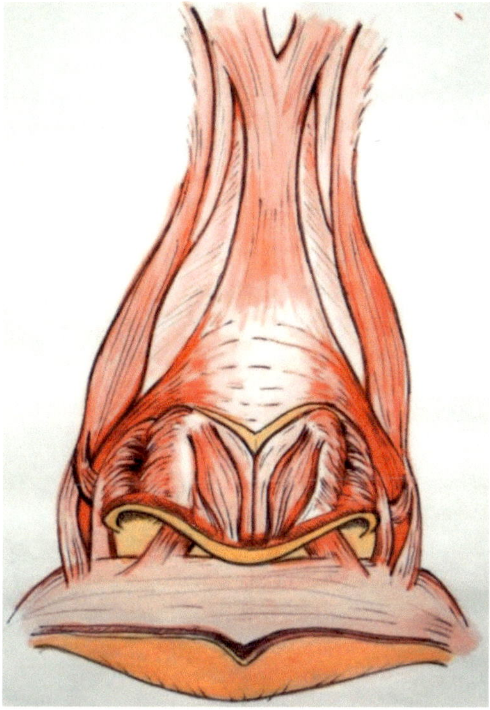

Figure 2. Nasal muscles. Front view.

Different authors have classified these muscles based on various criteria (Figs. 2 and 3). Aiach and Levignac [2] classify them according to the level of insertion in relation to the nostrils: above or below. Griesman [3] uses a physiological criterion, dividing them in elevators, depressors, dilators, and constrictors:

- Elevators that shorten the nose and open the nostrils:
  - *Procerus*
  - *Levator labii superioris alaeque nasi*
  - *Anomalus nasi*
- Depressors that enlarge the nose and open nostrils:
  - *Alar nasalis (dilator naris posterior)*
  - *Depressor septi nasi*
- Compressors that enlarge the nose and stretch nostrils:
  - *Transverse nasalis*
  - *Compressor narinum minor*
- Dilators:

- *Dilator naris anterior*

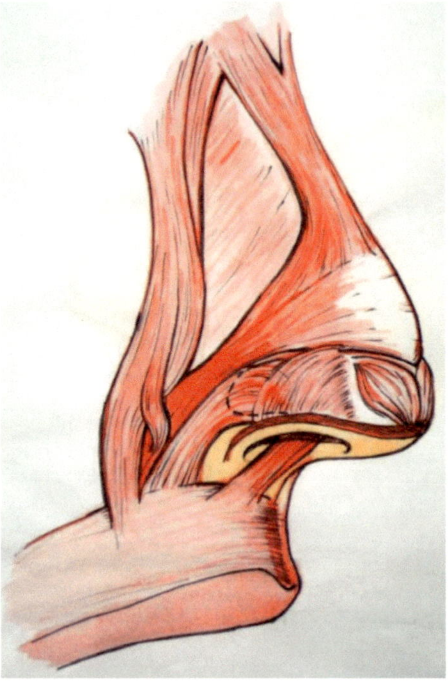

Figure 3. Nasal muscles. Lateral view.

The *procerus* originates in the *transverse nasalis* aponeurosis, nasal bones periosteum, and nasal lateral cartilage perichondrium, and ends in glabellar skin. As an elevator it antagonizes the *transverse nasalis* depressor action.

The *levator labii superioris alaeque nasi* originates in the medial portion of the *orbicularis oculi* and the frontal process of the maxilla, inserting down in the nasolabial fold, nasal ala, and skin and muscles of the upper lip. It has a nasal fascicle that covers the origin of the *transverse nasalis*. The main function is to elevate the nasal ala and open the nostrils.

The *anomalus* originates in the frontal process of the maxilla inserting in nasal bones, nasal lateral cartilage, the *procerus*, and the *transverse nasalis*. It is present in 50% of the population.

The *alar nasalis,* also known as *dilator naris posterior,* originates in the maxilla over the lateral incisor and inserts in the nasal ala. This muscle opens the nostrils.

The *depressor septi nasi* originates in the nasal spine of the maxilla inserting in the membranous septum and medial crus of alar cartilages. The contraction of this muscle turns downward the nasal tip. According to Zide [4], there are some superficial fibers that originate in the *orbicularis oris,* and insert in the columella, which are responsible for the elevation of the lip as the nasal tip turns down.

http://dx.doi.org/10.5772/62070

The *transverse nasalis* originates in the maxilla above the incisor fossa, sharing some fibers with the *levator labi superioris alaeque nasi,* then it inserts in an aponeurosis over the nasal dorsum, joining with the contralateral muscle. The contraction of this muscle stretches the nasal vestibule by descending the lateral crus of the alar cartilage.

The *compressor narinum minor* is a small muscle that descends from the nasal lateral cartilage to the skin over the nostrils. It is present in 57% of the population. Superficial to this muscle is the *dilator naris anterior,* whose main function is to open the nostrils. This is a fan-shaped muscle that originates in the nasal lateral cartilage and the *transverse nasalis* and inserts in the caudal border of the lateral crus of the alar cartilage and in nostrils skin. The contraction of this muscle can be felt by compressing the nasal ala between two fingers.

2. Botulinum toxin properties

Clostridium Botulinum are bacteria that produce different types of toxins. Seven types have been identified, known as A, B, C, D, E, F, and G. They all produce denervation and atrophy of muscles. The most powerful is toxin A, being the elective treatment of many dystonias. Type B is also available for medical use; it has a faster but shorter effect (Myobloc ®).

We refer to our experience with toxin A commercialized by Allergan with the name BOTOX® (other products differ in pharmacodynamics and pharmacokinetics).

3. Toxin handling

Botulinum toxin is commercialized as crystallized powder that contains 100 UI per vial. Reconstitution should be done with sterile, preservative-free saline solution. The product final concentration depends on the volume used for reconstitution. For cosmetic use in the nasal area, reconstitution of the toxin is recommended to be done with 1 ml of saline solution per vial. This avoids diffusion to neighboring muscles, preventing undesired effects.

The manufacturer recommends the use within 4 HS after reconstitution, but experience has demonstrated that the reconstituted solution does not loose effectiveness if conserved in a refrigerator at 4°C.

We like to use 0.3 ml syringes with 30 G needle (Ultrafine II. Becton Dickinson-BD) for precise application. These syringes do not have dead space so no solution is lost and allows a better dosage, a fundamental aspect in the nasal area.

Botulinum toxin can be injected intramuscular, subcutaneous, or intracuticular. Anesthetic cream can be applied locally if the patient is oversensitive. Other way to reduce pain is using cold packs.

4. Side effects and precautions

In patients with neuromuscular diseases such as myasthenia gravis or amyotrophic lateral sclerosis, it is relatively contraindicated. Application should be avoided during pregnancy and lactation. Drug interaction is limited to aminoglycosides, with which a lower dose is recommended. Most secondary effects are due to toxin diffusion to neighboring muscles. This is preventable using correct doses and injection planes. There are no long-term effects described with the toxin. With repeated application the effect can diminish, probably due to antitoxin antibodies.

5. Dosage and frequency

The clinical effect of the toxin starts between the second and the fourth day, and regularly lasts for four or five months. Generally, patients that are happy with the result come back to repeat the application when the effect starts to diminish. Stronger muscles require higher doses. When working in small areas, to prevent diffusion to neighboring muscles, reconstitution with lower volumes of saline solution is recommended. As a general rule, the limit per application per session is 400 UI, doses that are only used for spastic paralysis. In the nasal region, doses never exceed 20 UI.

6. Nasal application

6.1. Nasoglabellar wrinkles and bunny lines

Over the lateral wall of the nasal bridge an important percentage of the population have diagonal lines that go toward the nasal ala. This has been the first indication of BOTOX® in the nasal area suggested by Carruthers [5].

These wrinkles or bunny lines can be primary or secondary. The secondary ones, also known as BOTOX® effect, appear after the treatment with toxin in the glablellar muscles. That is why when treating frown wrinkles it is important to advert to patients the possibility of developing compensatory nasoglabellar wrinkles. This compensatory effect develops mostly in women that already have an insinuation of these wrinkles and have an outdoor life, which generates muscle contraction by sun exposure. By blocking frown muscles some people start contracting involuntarily the *nasalis transverse*. Primary wrinkles are frequent in people that gesticulate a lot, users of heavy glasses, chronic rhinitis, and those with clear eyes that try to close the lids in response to sun or light. These muscles get hypertrophied and hyperfunctional by forced and constant contraction, provoking wrinkles in the thin skin that covers them. They are more frequent in Caucasian people, and they get accentuated when they smile, talk, or get angry. Men have a thicker skin, thus having fewer wrinkles.

In patients with previous rhinoplasty, Botulinum toxin clinical effect is less evident, probably due to anatomic changes and muscular scar provoked by surgery.

It is important to differentiate wrinkles provoked by the *transverse nasalis* (described above) from wrinkles provoked by the *procerus*. The latter are horizontal lines that appear in the nasal root when the glabellar skin is pulled down by the contraction of the *procerus*. By eliminating both these wrinkles, a juvenile and relaxed appearance is obtained in the mid face. When we do not treat simultaneously the nasoglabellar and the glabellar wrinkles, the untreated ones develop compensatory contraction, producing a strange effect on nasal image.

Tamura [6] pointed out that in 40% of patients, the nasoglabellar wrinkles can be treated with 3 UI injected in each nasal wall in the muscular body. The other 60% of the patients present different patterns of muscular contraction, needing additional 2 UI in neighboring areas. He identifies three patterns of wrinkles that appear within the first 4 weeks of application: nasoalar, nasoorbicular, and nasociliar. The nasoalar lines are produced by the contraction of the alar fibers of the *levator labii superioris* and must be treated just over the nasal ala. The nasoorbicular and the nasociliar are produced by the contraction of the *orbicularis oculi*.

We inject 2–4 UI of Botulinum toxin in the *transverse nasalis* belly where it goes over the nasal bone. Then we observe the evolution, and if necessary perform the corrections following Tamura's recommendation.

6.1.1. Precaution

It is important to inject above the nasofacial groove to prevent diffusion of toxin to the *levator labii superioris*, causing lip ptosis and lip asymmetry. This can cause incompetence of the labial sphincter, creating problems to eat and talk.

Less frequent, but not less important complication is toxin diffusion to the *orbicularis oculi*, diminishing the pump effect over the lacrimal sac causing tearing. Diffusion to the *medial rectus* of the eye has been described, causing blurred vision.

It is important to avoid injecting the product in the angular artery, which can cause thrombosis and blindness.

To prevent these complications that are mainly caused by diffusion to neighboring muscles, and for which there is no antidote, it is preferable to avoid any kind of massage in the area after applying the toxin.

6.2. Nasal tip ptosis

As people age, the nasal tip tends to turn downward partially by the gravity forces and partially caused by the hyperkinetic action of the *depressor septi nasi* muscle over the caudal portion of the nasal septum. When this occurs, appearance turns senile, evil, and witch-like.

The importance of the *depresor septi nasi* in rhinoplasty has been remarked upon many years ago. Wright [7] in 1976 noted that a hyperactive muscle contributed to the tip ptosis, and that this phenomenon could be diagnosed by the "smile test." In 1983, Ham [8] reported that the *depressor septi nasi* was responsible for the tension in nasal tip and dorsum, and he recommended this muscle transection to solve the problem. Cachay-Velazquez [9, 10] described in 1992 the "rhino-gingivo-labial syndrome of the smile." He points out the importance of dynamic examining of face, which can reveal aesthetic imperfections, not so evident at rest. The rhino-gingivo-labial syndrome of the smile includes:

- Nasal tip ptosis
- Elevation and shortening of the superior lip
- Increased exposure oral mucosa

The author attributes this syndrome to the *depressor septi nasi* hypertrophy. For the correction he proposes excision of the *depressor septi nasi*, and a partial excision of *orbicularis oris* and *nasalis* muscles through a stab incision. There are no cases of nasal obstruction in the clinical experience of the author, contrary to what Converse [11] revealed about the importance of conserving this muscle.

De Souza Pinto [12] reported his technique called "dynamic rhinoplasty." He uses a Z-plasty based on the labial bridle and combines relaxation of the medial fascicle of the *depresor septi nasi*, with horizontal or vertical plication of the intermediate fascicle, depending on the length of the superior lip.

The nasal tip ptosis generally coincides with a short superior lip, entity described by Rohrich [13] as the functional unity of the inferior third of the nose. The *depressor septi nasi* and the *levator labii superioris alaeque nasi* are responsible for the muscular forces affecting this area in the dynamic and static models. The *depressor septi nasi* is sometimes considered as part of the *dilator naris*, muscle that originates in the incisor fossa of the maxilla, just below the *orbicularis oris*, and in the mucosa of the superior lip. The *depressor septi nasi* pulls down the nasal septum and ala stretching the nostrils. The interdigitation of this muscle with *dilator naris* is present in a small percentage of the population. In these cases, a paradoxical opening of the nostrils is provoked when these muscles contract together.

Due to anatomical variations described above and the multifactorial etiology of the nasal tip ptosis, BOTOX® application will have positive results only when the main cause of the defect is the muscular action. To evaluate the muscular strength it is important to observe the functional unity of the inferior third of the nose during forced smile. With this observation, we can predict which patients will have a good result with toxin. To perform the procedure we have to pull down the patient's upper lip over the teeth in order to open the nasolabial angle. In this way we elongate the muscle, making easier the identification of the muscle insertion in the base of the columella, where the needle should be introduced to inject 2–4 UI in the subcutaneous to avoid diffusion to the *orbicularis oris* (Fig. 4). If we are in the presence of a strong muscle, additional 2 UI can be used in the mid columella. In patients with interdigitation of the *depressor septi nasi* and the *dilator naris*, additional 4–5 UI are recommended in the nasal ala dorsum, inside the *dilator naris*, in order to obtain a better tip projection.

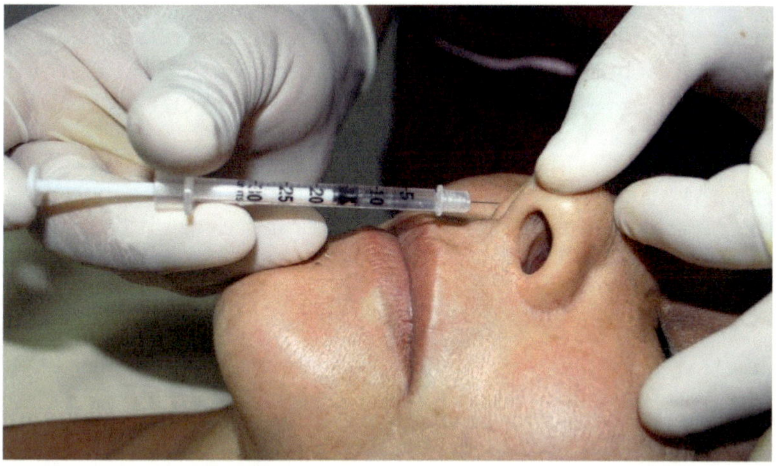

Figure 4. Application in the depressor septi nasi.

Peres Atamoros [14] created a therapeutic protocol that allows measuring of the tip elevation when using BOTOX®. He establishes that for a soft elevation, 2 UI must be injected in each *dilator naris* and 2 UI in the *depressor septi nasi* (total of 6 UI). For a medium elevation, 4 UI should be injected in each point (total of 12 UI). Finally, for a strong elevation 6 UI should be injected in each point (total of 18 UI).

In some patients, the use of BOTOX® increases the distance between the columellar base and the vermilion border, creating the appearance of a fuller and voluminous lip. It can also correct the gingival smile. If the toxin diffuses laterally in the base of the columella, it can affect the *levator labii superioris* and the *orbicularis oris*, provoking an unaesthetic elongation of the superior lip, filtrum flattening, and labial sphincter incompetence when talking and drinking.

The use of high doses in the nasal tip can produce an exaggerated opening of the nostrils and a strong elevation of the tip, leaving an unattractive appearance in the frontal view. The clinical effect in this area usually lasts for a shorter time than other parts of the face. The first days after the injection, the patient can experience pain in the nasal tip.

In order to obtain satisfactory results in nasal tip ptosis correction, it is important to understand the mechanism of the downward rotation of the tip when smiling. This mechanism depends on a functional unity with three components:

1. Cartilage frame (alar and accessory cartilages acting as a unique structure)
2. Muscle engine (*depressor septi nasi* and *levator labii superioris alaeque nasi*)
3. Neighboring structures (piriform fossa, valvular mechanism between the lateral and alar cartilages, areolar tissue of nasal dorsum and membranous septum)

BOTOX® application does not replace surgery in patients with static nasal tip ptosis, but it is useful in dynamic ptosis and in other defects caused by a hypertrophic or hyperactive *depressor septi nasi*, and with patients that do not desire a rhinoplasty. Besides, BOTOX® can be used temporarily in patients that are evaluating a surgical procedure. The application of toxin is a great combination with other minimal invasive procedures as bioplasty, fillers, and nasal rein. It is possible to obtain a reduction of the dynamic nasal tip ptosis, a correction on the shortening of the superior lip, and apparent absence of philtrum by using BOTOX® (Allergan Inc. Irvine, California).

When the *depressor septi nasi* contracts the nasal tip descends, making more evident the nasal tip ptosis. According with the interdigitation of this muscle with the *orbicularis oris,* it is classified in three subtypes:

1. Type I: totally inserted in the *orbicularis oris* (62%)
2. Type II: inserted in the periosteum and partially in the *orbicularis oris* (22%)
3. Type III: rudimentary muscle or absent

The *levator labii superioris alaeque nasi* originates in the frontal process of the maxilla and inserts down in skin of the nasal ala and superior lip. Its action is to elevate the superior lip and nasal ala. When contracting, together with the *depressor septi nasi* they descend the nasal tip while ascending the nasal ala and superior lip, thus opening the nostrils. Their contraction also produces a horizontal wrinkle, which divides the philtrum, and oral mucosa exposure. Until the discovery of the Botulinum toxin, acting over these muscles was only possible through surgical procedures. Now we can, applying 5 UI in the *depressor septi nasi* and 3 UI in each *levator labii superioris alaeque nasi,* attenuate this muscle's action, diminishing tip ptosis during smile, leaving the alar insertion in a neutral position. Also, the nasal angle opens to 110–115°. Satisfaction index in patients is very high and we have not observed serious secondary effects as labial sphincter incompetence or problems with talking.

With Botulinum toxin we can:

1. Correct the balance between the tip and the lip
2. Elongate the superior lip
3. Create the appearance of superior lip fullness
4. Keep the rotation:projection proportion during movement
5. Preserve the motor and sensitive innervation of the superior lip

In patients where the nasal tip ptosis is mainly due to aging, the result of BOTOX® is not as good as in young people where the muscular hypertrophy plays a major role. Precaution should be taken with patients with long lips and little vermilion, since there is significant risk of lip ptosis after the procedure.

6.3. Nasal flutter

Some people, naturally or under stress (emotional or physical), present wide movements of nasal flutter that enlarge the nostrils. This nasal flutter can be very embarrassing. Generally, people with short and flat nasal bridge with wide nasal ala present more active nasal muscles, which allow them to voluntarily move the nasal ala. The widened nostrils can take different forms expressing in the face moods such as anger, fear, worry, fatigue, reprobation, or stress.

The nasal flutter is the result of involuntary and repeated contraction of the inferior portion of the *alar nasalis* muscle, also known as *dilator naris posterior*. This muscle originates in the maxilla over the lateral incisive, is medial to the *transverse nasalis* in the nasolabial sulcus, travels through the nasal ala, and inserts in the caudal portion of the alar cartilage and skin of the nostrils. The medial fibers can join the *depressor septi nasi*. Its main action is to move the nasal ala laterally and downward, opening the nostrils and preventing the ala collapse during inspiration.

The side of the columella and the septum turns visible when the nostrils open exaggeratedly. This unaesthetic appearance gets accentuated with the contraction of the *depressor septi nasi*. In people with wide nasal base and ability to move the nasal ala, a stretching effect is seen in nostrils after applying BOTOX® in the *dilator naris posterior*. The injection of 5–10 UI, bilaterally, in the area of greater contraction of the *dilator naris posterior* (over the nasal ala), has diminished the nasal flutter for 3–4 months (Fig. 5). We have not experienced secondary effects after the use of toxin in this area.

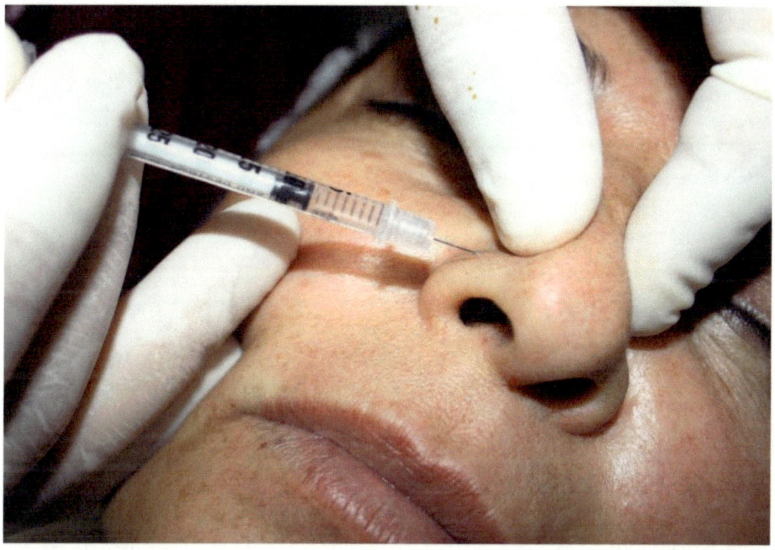

Figure 5. Application in the levator labii superioris alaeque nasi.

6.4. Botox® in nasal dorsum hyperhidrosis

Excessive sweating of the face generally affects areas as forehead, cheeks, scalp, lips, nasal dorsum, and ala. This is less frequent than axillary or hands and feet sweating but is highly detrimental for social and occupational life because it is extremely exposed to sight. Botulinum toxin blocks the liberation of acetylcholine in synapses that regulate the production of eccrine glands. The incidence of this disorder in the population is not known, but statistically it is more frequent in man and tends to worsen with aging. The permanent sweat impedes the correct application of creams, makeup, and sun block. And sometimes it makes glasses slide over the wet surface producing local irritation.

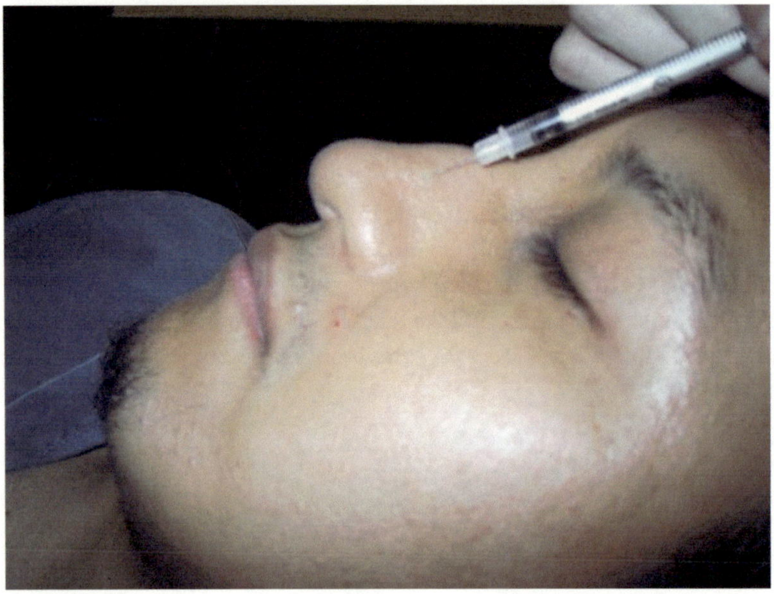

Figure 6. Application in nasal dorsum for hyperhidrosis

In some women, local sweating can appear in the premenopause together with the heat waves that characterize this period. Usually, these symptoms disappear spontaneously. Other stimuli for facial sweating are: caffeine, physical activity, stress, seasoned food, and heat.

A precise diagnosis of the area of sweating can be made through the test of Minor (iodinated alcohol and starch).

To treat this disorder, injections must be intracuticular, producing skin whitening and papules, in order to act over glands and not over muscles. This is a painful procedure, so we recommend the use of anesthetic cream, or if the patient is oversensitive, a local nerve blocking for the nasal area. The dose is 1–2 UI per injection, with 1 cm space between them, until covering the whole area of hyperhidrosis (Figs. 6 and 7). It is important to conserve symmetry while working, in order to avoid asymmetry that can affect the muscles. The patient is called back at day 10 after injection to evaluate the results, and if any area is still sweating, it is corrected. The effects in general last for seven months.

6.5. Botox® in the treatment of multiple eccrine hidrocystoma

Eccrine hidrocystomas is a cystic lesion of sweat gland ducts described by Andrew Ross Robinson in 1983. Incidence is higher in women. Multiple eccrine hidrocystoma are papule-

http://dx.doi.org/10.5772/62070

cystic lesions of elevated surface with a blue coloration that is seen through a transparent dome, easily confused with blackheads. It is common to find them in the facial area surrounding the eyes, forehead, nose, and superior lip. The etiology is a defect in transpiration or insensible perspiration. If ruptured or spontaneously broken, a clear and transparent liquid drains. It is presented in literature as an infrequent disease, but we think that is because of ignorance and misdiagnose with blackhead. This condition worsens with transpiration and environmental humidity, thus enlarging in summer and reducing in winter.

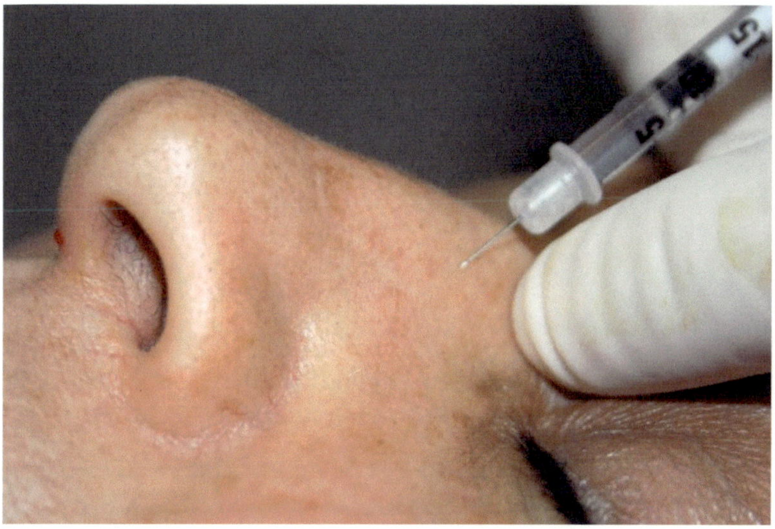

Figure 7. Application in nasal dorsum for hyperhidrosis pseudo-blackhead.

Based on our experience with botulinum toxin type A for the use of focal hyperhidrosis and the amount of bibliography about the effect of Botulinum toxin in parasympathetic fibers, we started using it in this disorder as well [15]. The application is similar to what is described above for hyperhidrosis. Results are excellent with complete reconstitution of the areas treated.

Author details

Diego Schavelzon[1*], Guillermo Blugerman[1], Gabriel Wexler[2] and Lorena Martinez[1]

*Address all correspondence to: drschavelzon@centrosbys.com

1 Plastic Surgery Department of Centros B&S, Buenos Aires, Argentina

2 Universidad Nacional del Nordeste, Argentina

Conflict of interest

The authors declare no conflict of interest.

Informed consent was obtained from the patients included in the chapter.

References

[1] Letourneau, A., and Daniel, R. K. The superficial musculoaponeurotic system of the nose. *Plast. Reconstr. Surg.* 1988 ;82(1):48-57.

[2] Aiach, G., and Levignac, J. La Rhinoplastie Esthetique. Paris: Masson edit. 1986;13-14.

[3] Griesman, B. Muscles and cartilages of the nose from the standpoint of a typical rhinoplasty. *Arch. Otolaryngol.* 1944: 39:334.

[4] Zide B.M. Nasal Anatomy: The muscles and tip sensation. *Aesthetic. Plast. Surg.* 1985; 9(3):193-196.

[5] Carruthers J., and Carruthers A. Practical cosmetic BOTOX techniques. *J. Cutan. Med Surg.* 1999 Dec; 3 Suppl 4:S49-S52.

[6] Tamura B.M., Odo M.Y., Chang B., *et al.* Treatment of nasal wrinkles with botulinum toxin. *Dermatol Surg.* 2005;31(3):271-275.

[7] Wright, W.K. Symposium: The supra-tip in rhinoplasty – A dilemma: II. Influence of surrounding structure and prevention. *Laryngoscope.* 1976;86(1):50-52.

[8] Ham, K.S., Chung, S.C., and Lee, S.H. Complications of oriental augmentation rhinoplasty. *Ann. Acad. Med. Singapore.* 1983;12(2 Suppl):460-462.

[9] Cachay-Velasquez, H., and Laguinge, R. Aesthetic treatment of the columella. *Ann. Plast. Surg.* 1989;22(5):370-379.

[10] Cachay-Velasquez, H. Rhinoplasty and facial expression. *Ann. Plast. Surg.* 1992 ;28(5): 427-433.

[11] Converse, J. M. (Ed.). *Plastic and Reconstructive Surgery.* Philadelphia: Saunders, 1964. pp. 702-703.

[12] De Souza Pinto, E.B., Da Rocha, R. P., Filho, W. Q., *et al.* Anatomy of the median part of the septum depressor muscle in aesthetic surgery. *Aesthetic Plast. Surg.* 1998;22(2): 111-115.

[13] Rohrich, Rod J. Importance of the depressor septi nasi muscle in rhinoplasty: Anatomic study and clinical application. *Plast. Reconstruct. Surg.* 2000;105(1):376-383; discussion 384-388.

[14] Benedetto, Anthony V. Botulinum toxin in clinical medicine. *Clin. Dermatol.* 2003;21(6):465-468.

[15] Blugerman G, and Schavelzon D. Multiple Eccrine Hidrocystomas: a new therapeutic option with Botulinum Toxin, *Dermatol. Surg.* 2003; 29(5):557-558.

Chapter 11

Five Fluorouracil, Hyaluronidase, and Triamcinolone in the Nasal Region

Guillermo Blugerman, Diego Schavelzon and Gabriel Wexler

Additional information is available at the end of the chapter

http://dx.doi.org/10.5772/62068

Abstract

Introduction: The use of five fluorouracil (5 FU) as antifibrotic started in the 1960s, in the hands of ophthalmologists, to prevent adherence after glaucoma and pterigion surgery. In 1999, Fitzpatrick presented his experience in keloids and hypertrophic scars, making a great contribution to their treatment. Fibroblasts' main function is collagen synthesis; in vicious scar the amount of collagen is normal, but what is altered is the ratio between collagen subtypes. The use of triamcinolone, the previous standard treatment, produced different degrees of atrophy and telangiectasias.

Technique: Infiltration is done in the center of fibrosis, weekly for the first month, then every 15 days until reaching the desired result. Softening, loss of volume and retraction are seen since the first session. Also pain and itching disappears.

Histopathology: Biopsy of treated scars has organized collagen fibers and less fibroblasts compared to nontreated scars.

Clinical applications: hypertrophic scars or keloids fixed to deep planes, "supratip" post-rhinoplasty fibrosis, post-rhinoplasty fibrosis (as preparation for other treatments), foreign body granulomas, and post-burn retractions. The use in supratip deformity when secondary to rhinoplasty fibrotic scar has proven very effective, and also as preparation for surgical (secondary rhinoplasty) and nonsurgical (bioplasty) procedures.

Conclusion: Our experience in the treatment of nasal scars, fibrosis, and retraction with 5 FU is favorable. The results of infiltration with 5FU, hyaluronidase and triamcinolone in low dose have clinical and histological demonstration of collagen synthesis reduction and reorganization of collagen cicatrizal fibers.

Keywords: Corticosteroids, fibrosis, fibrosis histopathology, fibrosis treatment, five fluorouracil, fibroblasts, foreign body granulomas, healing, hyaluronidase, hypertrophic scar, keloids, nasal aesthetics, nasal dermatology, nasal deformity, nasal reconstruction, post-rhinoplasty fibrosis, burn sequelae, scar, scarring disorders, supratip deformity

1. Introduction

Since Fitzpatrick [1] published his work with five fluorouracil (5FU) in 1999, we included it in our daily practice. The most frequent use of this drug is for treatment and prevention of hypertrophic scars, keloids, and foreign body granulomas [2].

The particular anatomy of the skin in each nasal subunit makes scarring process completely different among them (Fig. 1). The skin of the tip is thick, has follicular units, and sebaceous glands, whereas the dorsum skin is thin with almost no subcutaneous tissue. Because of these, the nasal tip skin reacts violently to injury, with an important inflammatory process and residual edema that generates unaesthetic deformities. The dorsum skin reacts softly to injuries, with light inflammation and scarring, but strong adherence to deep structures due to its thin composition. The etiologies of scarring in the nose are:

- Congenital (angioma)
- Traumatic
- Surgical
- Infectious
- Implants

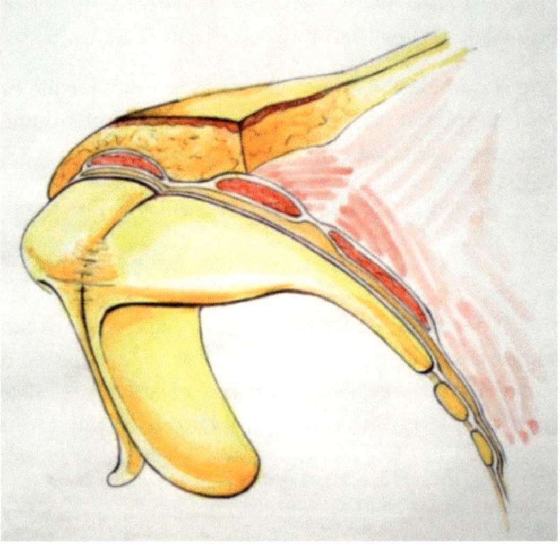

Figure 1. Anatomical structure of nasal tip and dorsum.

Fibroblasts' proliferation and migration play a major role in wound healing. Their main metabolic function is collagen, elastin, and proteoglycans synthesis. Fibroblasts' suppression in hypertrophic scars and keloids is essential since collagen synthesis is increased by 14% and 20%, respectively, compared to normal skin. Other studies show a higher amount of fibroblasts

http://dx.doi.org/10.5772/62068

without significant increase in collagen synthesis but with altered proportions between collagen I, III, and IV. These studies also show an increased production of fibronectin by fibroblasts. The local increase of collagenase inhibitors has also been reported.

Local steroids have been the gold standard treatment for nasal inflammatory and fibrotic processes for years, but its use has important side effects and complications. Triamcinolone usually generates different grades of skin atrophy and telangiectasias in the nasal tip and ala.

5 FU is a citostatic antimetabolite drug that inhibits cell proliferation by:

- Inhibition of thymidylate synthase avoiding DNA synthesis
- Incorporation in RNA and DNA altering its function
- Interference with glycosyltransferases altering cell membranes (Fig. 2)

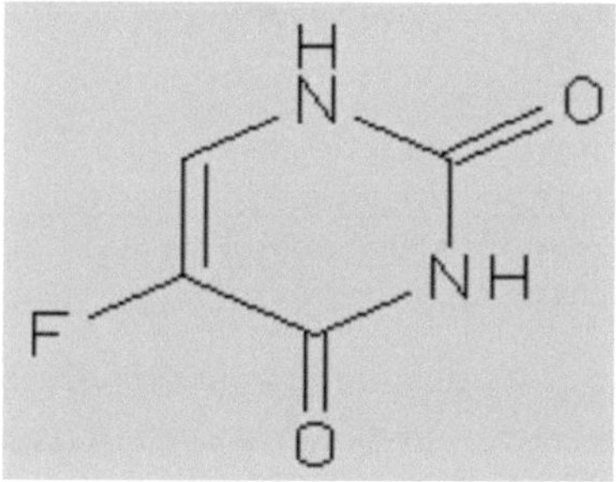

Figure 2. Molecular structure of 5 FU.

It has been proved in laboratory tests that 5 FU produces a slight reduction of collagen synthesis in normal fibroblasts but a drastic reduction in altered ones, as in Dupuytren illness [3]. Apparently, it also inhibits the collagen synthesis stimulation effect of TGF1 (transforming growth factor).

5 FU has been used for years in treatment of premalignant and malignant lesions of skin and mucosa due to its selective toxicity for dysplastic epithelium and fibroblasts. The first application of 5 FU was as an antifibrotic to prevent fibrous scarring after glaucoma surgery and to avoid relapse in pterigion surgery in the 1960s [4, 5, 6, 7, 8, 9]. In February of 1999, its use was reported to prevent fibrous adherence after tendon reconstructive surgery. One month after Fitzpatrick published his 7-year experience of over a thousand patients with 5 FU in hypertrophic scars and keloids. This magnificent work encouraged our team to include it in our office with positive results. Since Lambros published his work in 2004 [10], our team also added hyaluronidase. This last is an enzyme that increases connective tissue permeability by hyaluronic acid hydrolysis. Hyaluronic acid is a polysaccharide of connective tissue and other specialized tissues as the umbilical cord and the vitreous humor. Hydrolysis is done between the C1of glucosamine and C4 of glucuronic acid. This reduces temporarily the intercellular cement viscosity, promoting diffusion of injected solution, exudates, and transudates facilitating absorption.

Triamcinolone is a steroid; it diffuses through cell membranes binding with cytoplasmic receptors that are translocated to the nucleus generating the transcription of proteins that are responsible for their effects. It reduces tissue response to inflammation, reducing it symptoms without treating the specific cause. To do this it reduces the white blood cell (WBC) migration to the affected tissue. The most important effects are:

- Inhibition of phagocytosis
- Inhibition of liberation of lysosomal enzymes and inflammatory mediators
- Reduction of capillary permeability and WBC adhesion to capillary endothelium
- Reduction of blood concentration of T-cells, eosinophils, and monocytes
- Reduction of immunoglobulin binding with cellular receptors

In the past 14 years, we have been using a preparation of 5FU, hyaluronidase, and triamcinolone for the nasal area, and we have not had the complications and side effects observed with steroids monotreatment.

2. Technique

5 FU (Fluorouracil- Filaxis 500mg) is presented commercially as ampoules of 10 ml containing 50 mg per ml. Triamcinolone (Kenacort-A-BSM) is used in its acetonide form of 40mg/ml and is commercialized in ampoules of 1ml (Fig. 3). Hyluronidase (Unidasa Roux Ocefa) is commercialized in ampoules that contain 500 UI of testicular ovine freeze-dried powder hyaluronidase. We use 2.7 ml of 5 FU and 0.3ml of triamcinolone to reconstitute hyaluronidase (5 FU solution). For the application, a 0.3 or 0.5 ml Luer lock syringe and 30 G needle are preferred. This allows a better dosage and correct plane of infiltration. We have never used more that 0.5 ml of the solution in the nasal area per session. The infiltration is done with multiple punctures in the "heart" of the fibrotic lesion. In the first month, one session is done per week; then it is spaced to every fifteen days. The improvement is evaluated with three parameters: hardening reduction, loss of volume, and reduction of cutaneous retraction. Positive changes are observed since the first session, not only in the above parameters but also in aesthetics and pain–itching symptomatology. Some cases are complemented with kinesiology treatment in order to obtain a better functional and cosmetic result.

3. Histopathology

If after finishing the treatment a surgical procedure was needed to improve the result, the surgical piece was sent to the pathologist and compared to nontreated scarring tissue resections. Results informed reduction of fibrosis and rearrangement of collagen tissue in the treated pieces. These results are illustrated in the images. In the tissue of the right side of the scar proliferation of fibrous tissue, great amount of fibroblasts and collagen fibers forming tangles

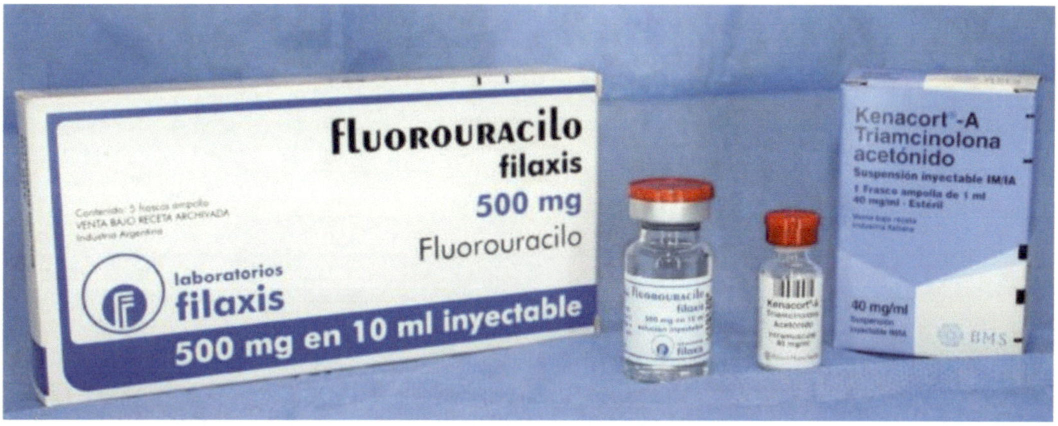

Figure 3. Commercial presentations of 5 FU and triamcinolone

is seen (Fig. 4). In the tissue of the left, treated with 5 FU solution, there are less fibroblasts, and the collagen fibers adopt a parallel disposition (Fig. 5).

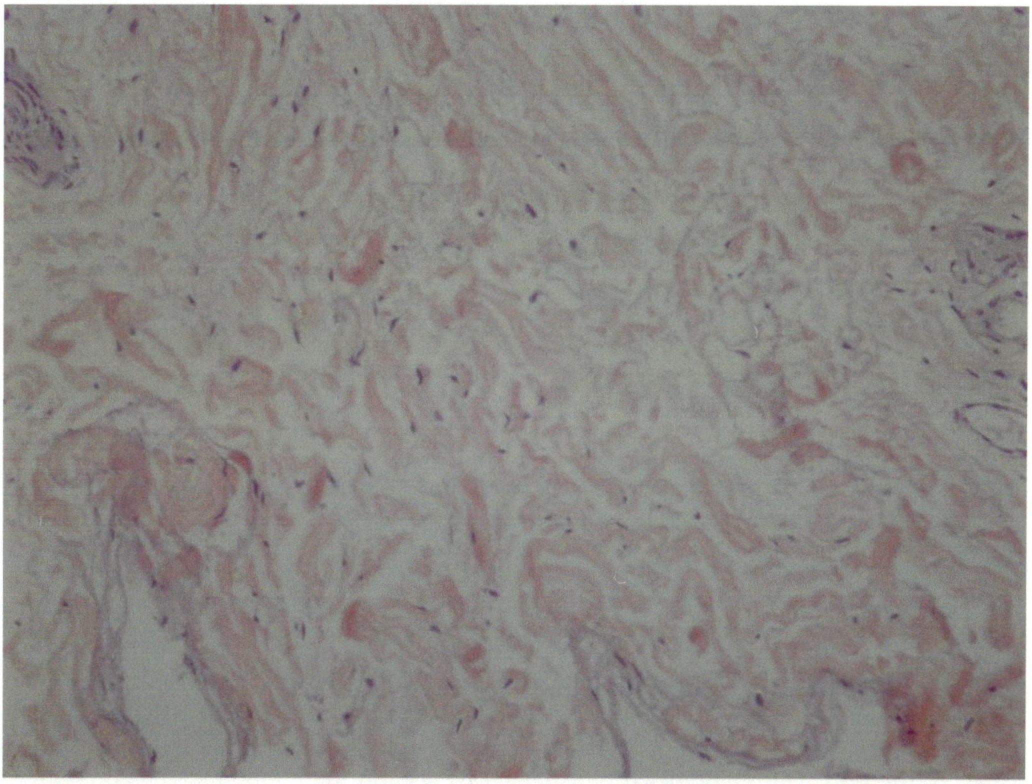

Figure 4. Microscopic image of fibrosis without any infiltration treatment (left).

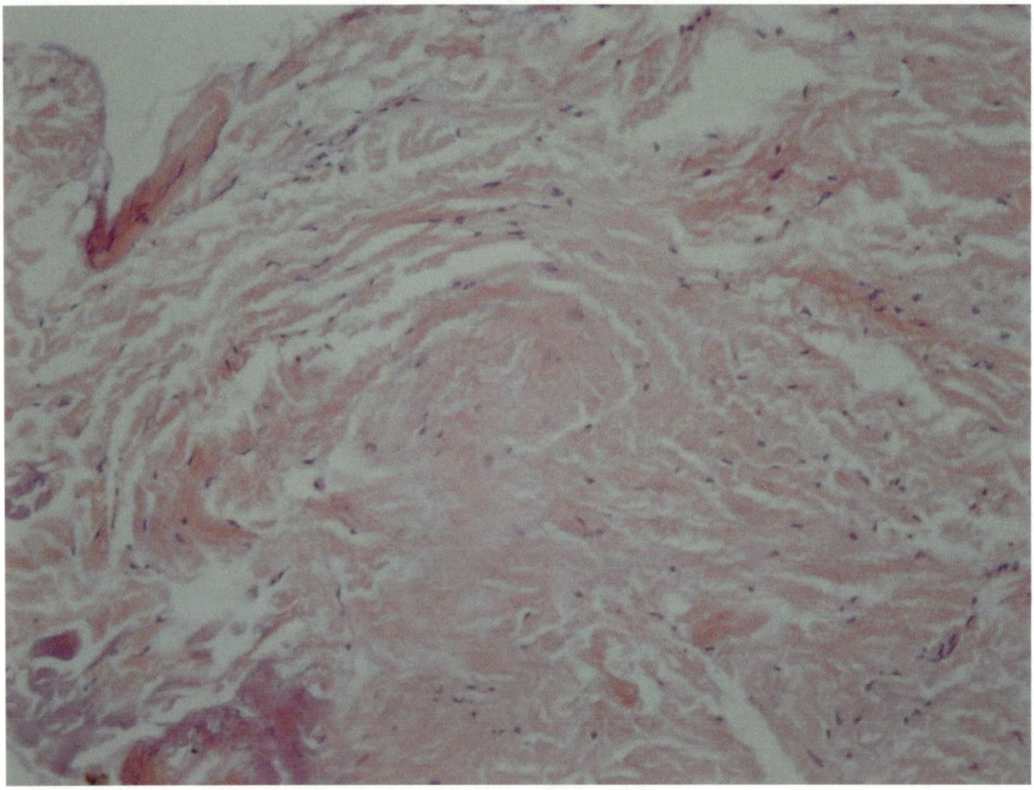

Figure 5. Microscopic image of fibrosis after infiltration with 5 FU (right).

4. Clinical applications

- Hypertrophic scars or keloids fixed to deep planes
- "Supratip" post-rhinoplasty fibrosis
- Post-rhinoplasty fibrosis (as preparation for other treatments)
- Foreign body granulomas
- Post-burn retractions

4.1. Hypertrophic scars or keloids fixed to deep planes

The nose, being a mid-facial and projected structure, is exposed to trauma that leaves scarring sequels in the skin. Traumatic scarring if healed by second intention generates unaesthetic scars. The use of 5 FU, triamcinolone, and hyaluronidase for hypertrophic scars and keloids in the nasal area is in our hands more effective and safe than the use of steroids alone. When these scars are fixed to deep planes, the infiltration is done as preparation to subcision and then a filler as Polymethylmetacrilate (PMMA) is used to prevent the relapse of the adherence (Figs. 6 and 7).

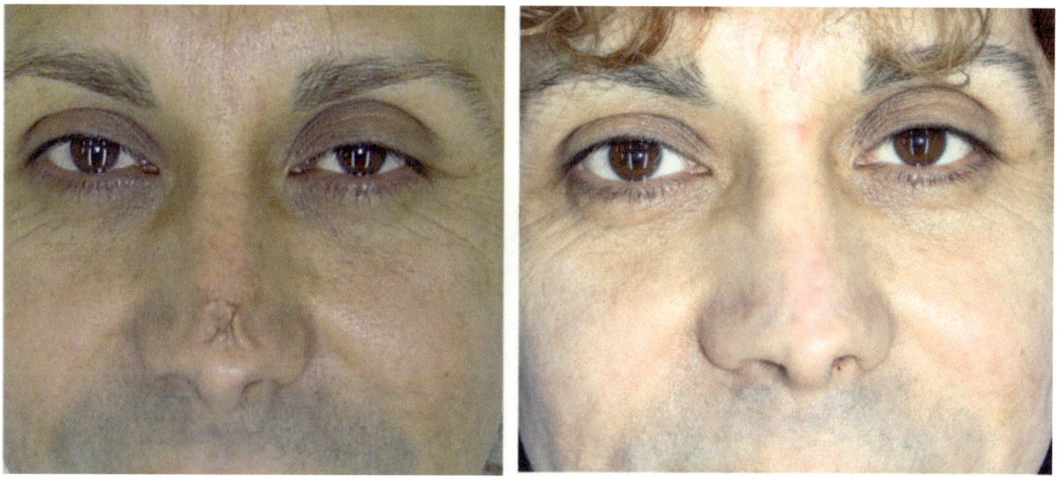

Figure 6. Nasal tip scar after cartilage graft infection and extrusion. Frontal view before and after 5 FU injection and dermabration.

4.2. "Supratip" post-rhinoplasty fibrosis

One of the most frequent complications of rhinoplasty is the healing fibrosis that is formed over time, known as "fibrous supratip." It can be the result of a badly executed rhinoplasty or defective healing process. It is very frequent among beginners and even experts still have this complication. There are many causes of supratip deformity and each demands a specific treatment. Bahman Guyuron [11] conducted a clinical and histological study to unmask the surgical causes of this deformity. This study shows that clinical supratip is observed in 9% of primary and 36% of secondary consults of rhinoplasty. In primary cases, the deformity is the result of: tip inadequate projection, caudal dorsum overprojection, lateral inferior cartilages cephalic orientation, or a combination of these. In secondary cases, the deformity is the result of: subcorrection or overcorrection of caudal dorsum, overresection of medial valve, subprojected tip, or a combination of these. The histophatological study of the supratip soft tissue demonstrated significant fibrosis in 14 of 16 secondary patients and 13 of 23 primary patients. The supratip deformity can be avoided through appropriate resection of caudal dorsum (in order not to leave dead space), nasal tip projection, and joining with stitches the subcutaneous tissue over the cartilages in the supratip area. When diagnosed early, if the tip has adequate projection and the supratip tissue can be collapsed by pressure, the elective treatment is compressive tape. If after 6 weeks the response is not positive, 0.2–0.4 ml of 5 FU solution is injected in the deep (Figs. 8 and 9) subcutaneous tissue. This infiltration can be repeated monthly until reaching the desired result. (The judicious use of 5 FU solution can help in most supratip deformities caused by fibrosis when the caudal septum and the tip cartilages are strong. If the cartilaginous frame is weak, infiltration will not solve the problem.)

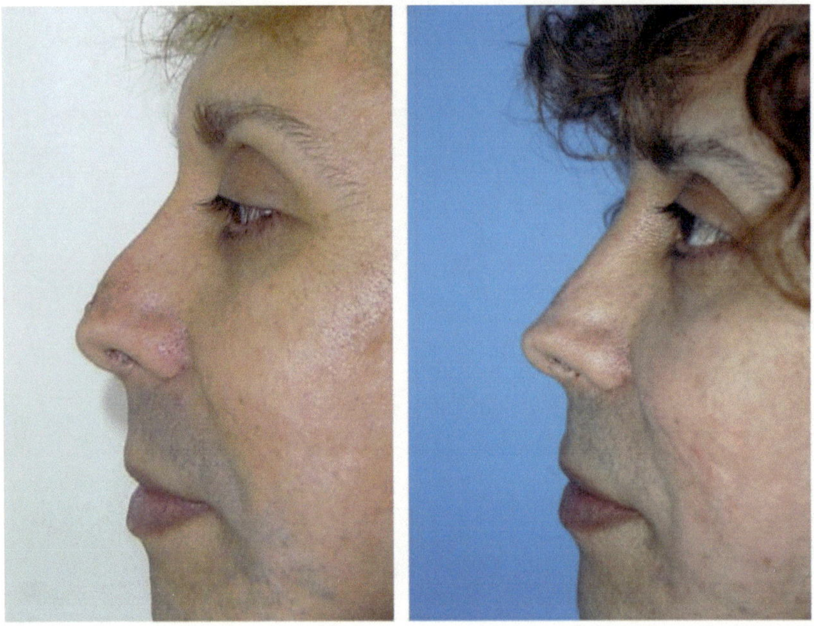

Figure 7. Nasal tip scar after cartilage graft infection and extrusion. Lateral view before and after 5 FU injection and dermabration.

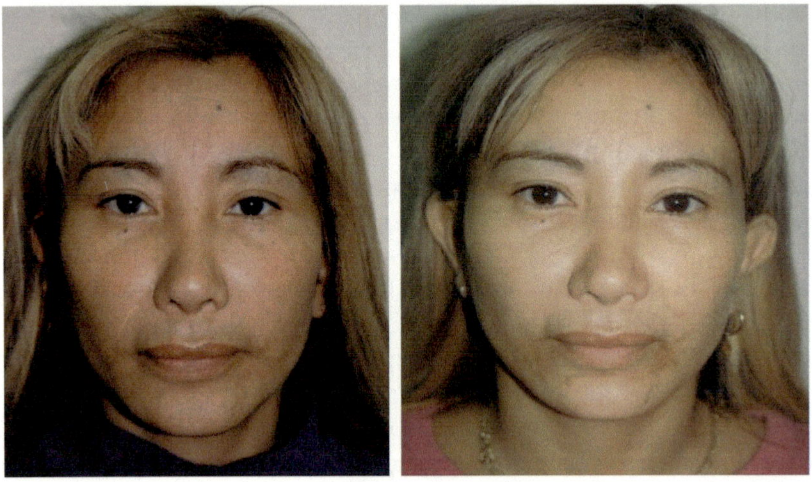

Figure 8. Fibrose supratip after previous procedure solve after 5 year with 0.3 ml of 5 FU single injection. Frontal view.

Infiltration can reduce a big supratip to a small one but with an important risk of skin atrophy.

Other authors such as Gruber [12] prefer to start with infiltration after 4–6 weeks of surgery, when most edema has disappeared. He uses 1–2 mg of triamcinolone (0.1–0.2 cc of triamcinolone 10 mg/cc) in the supratip or other fibrous area. Pastorek [13] uses small steroids doses during and immediately after surgery, having excellent results in his hands. If a severe supratip deformity is the consequence of inadequate cartilage resection or subprojection of the tip, a surgical correction or bioplasty is needed. Sheen [14] suggested in 1979 that most supratip deformities were caused by caudal dorsum overresection. He proposed then the use of cartilage graft to correct this deformity.

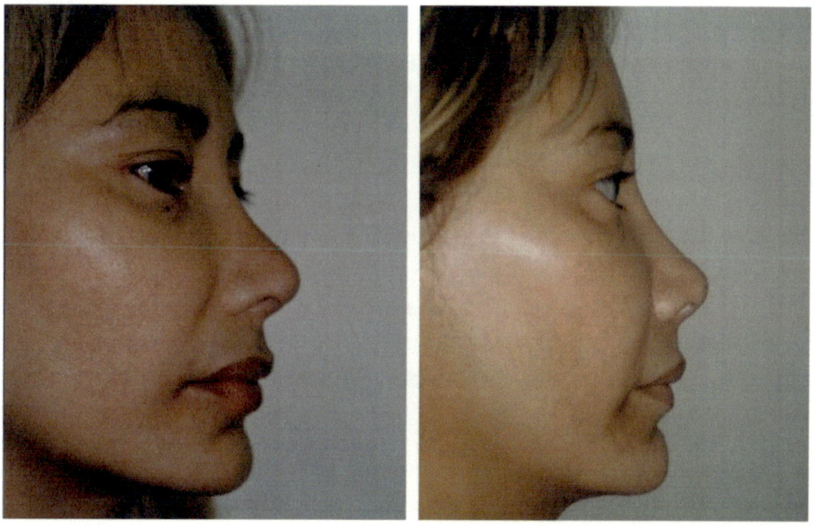

Figure 9. Fibrose supratip after previous procedure solved after 5 years with 0.3 ml of 5 FU single injection. Frontal view. Lateral view.

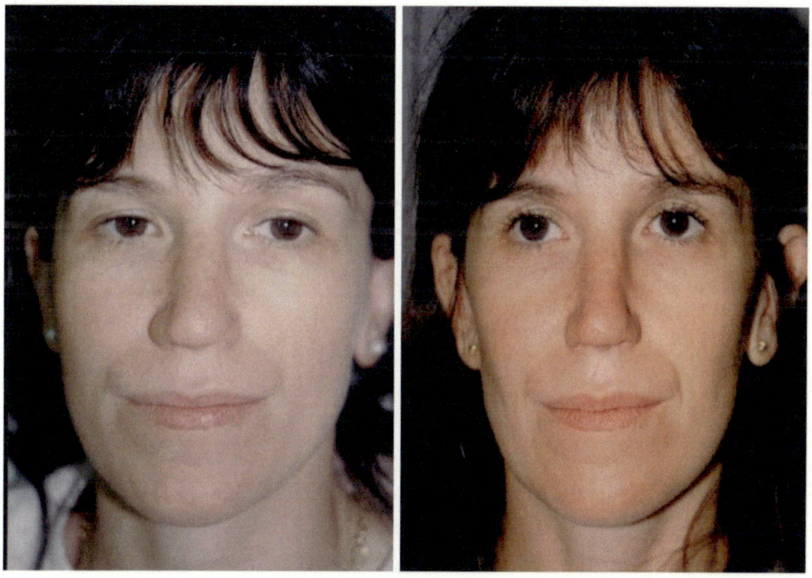

Figure 10. Patient with 3 previous rhinoplasties. Three applications of 5 FU solution were done.

Nowadays, it is widely accepted that healing fibrotic tissue formed to fill the dead space is the most frequent cause of supratip deformity post-rhinoplasty. But it was not until Guyuron's work that this was scientifically confirmed.

4.3. Post-rhinoplasty fibrosis, as preparation for other treatments

After several surgical procedures, the nose can be involved in different grades of fibrosis, turning the skin hard and inelastic. Before performing a secondary rhinoplasty or a bioplasty, we prefer preparing the area with some applications of the 5 FU solution, in order to soften the tissue (Fig. 10).

4.4. Foreign body granulomas

The use of fillers in the nasal area is a very popular method to correct slight deformities. There are many different materials and each of them produces a different degree of fibrotic reaction in the tissue. In most cases, this is a controlled reaction and leads to the expected result. But in some cases, an overreaction of patient immune system, bad application technique, or the chemistry of the material used provoke the formation of foreign body granulomas, resulting in unaesthetic deformities.

The use of triamcinolone in these cases can generate skin atrophy, thus turning the deformity more visible. When the filler used is hyaluronic acid, pure hyaluronidase should be infiltrated as stated by Brody [15] and Hirsch [16]. Infiltration is done with 100 UI in the area of hyaluronic acid excess (Fig. 11). This dissolves the acid, solving the fibrosis. When alloplastic materials were used, we preferred the 5 FU solution for infiltration because it does not have the side effects of steroids monotreatment. The application has a double effect, the pharmacological effect of the drugs, and the mechanical effect of disruption by the fluid pressure.

4.5. Post-burn retractions

The nasal skin usually gets affected in facial burns. The scarring retraction can deform the tip, ala, or both, stretching the nostrils. We use the 5 FU solution infiltration in these fibrous areas in order to increase the tissue elasticity and prepare them for secondary procedures as PMMA bioplasty or compound auricular graft.

5. Complications

The use of 5 FU solution, in young patients mostly, can cause tissue necrosis. This is relatively frequent in keloid treatment, resulting in ulcers or brown stains in the application spots. However, in the nasal region we have not observed this complication, mainly because of the low dosage. In this way, by using a progressive treatment instead of an aggressive one, side effects are kept to the minimum.

http://dx.doi.org/10.5772/62068

6. Conclusions

Through this chapter, we have presented our experience in the treatment of scars, fibrosis, retractions, and deformities over the nasal skin. The results of our 14-year experience with 5 FU solution (5 FU, triamcinolone, and hyaluronidase) have the histopathological demonstration of effectiveness in collagen fibers synthesis reduction and fiber rearrangement, thus explaining the positive clinical effect.

Author details

Guillermo Blugerman[1*], Diego Schavelzon[1] and Gabriel Wexler[2]

*Address all correspondence to: blugerman@centrosbys.com

1 Plastic Surgery Department of Centros ByS,Centros B&S de Excelencia en Cirugía Plástica, Argentina

2 Universidad Nacional del Nordeste, Argentina

Conflict of interest
The Authors declare no conflict of interest.
Informed consent was obtained from patients included in the chapter.

References

[1] Fitzpatrick R. Treatment of inflamed hypertrophic scars using intralesional 5-FU. *Dermatol Surg*. 1999;25(3):224-232.

[2] Blugerman G. Keloids and Hipertrofic scars. Congreso de Cirugía Plástica del Cono Sur, Porto Alegre, Brasil, Mayo 2001.

[3] Jemec, B., C. Linge, et al. The effect of 5-fluorouracil on Dupuytren fibroblast proliferation and differentiation. *Chir Main* 2000;19(1):15-22.

[4] Blugerman G., Schavelzon D. Intralesional use of 5-FU in subcutaneous fibrosis. *J. Drugs Dermatol*. 2003; 2: 169-171

[5] Yamamoto T., Varani J., Soong H.K., Lichter P.R. Effect of 5-fluorouracil and mitomycin on cultured rabbit subconjunctival fibroblast. *Ophthalmology* 1990;97:1202-1210.

[6] Yeatts R.P., Ford J.G., Stanton C.A., Reed J.W. Topical 5-fluorouracil in the intra epithelial neoplasia of the conjuntiva and cornea. *Ophthalmology* 1995; 102:1388-1344.

[7] Lee D.A., Shapourifar-Tehrani S., Kitada S. The effect of 5-fluorouracil and cytarabine on human fibroblasts from Tenon's capsule. *Invest Ophthalmol Vis Sci.* 1990;31:1848-1855.

[8] Schellini Silvana A. Uso do 5-fluorouracil no intra-operatório da cirurgia do pterígio. *Arq Bras Oftalmol.* 2000 63(2): 111-114.

[9] Acali Augustine et al. Decrease in adhesión formation by a single application of 5Fluorouracil after flexor tendon injury. *Plast Reconstr Surg.*1999;103(1):151-158.

[10] Lambros V. The use of hyaluronidase to reverse the effects of hyaluronic acid filler. *Plast Reconstr Surg.* 2004; 114(1):277.

[11] Guyuron, Bahman. Supratip deformity: A closer look. *Plast Reconstr Surg.* 2000.105(3):1140-1151.

[12] Gruber, Ronald P. MD. Supratip deformity: A closer look by Bahman Guyuron, MD, Louis DeLuca, MD, and Richard Lash, MD. *Plast Reconstr Surg.* 2000 105(3): 1152-1153.

[13] Pastorek, N. Surgery of the Nasal Tip. Presented at the Dallas Rhinoplasty Symposium, Dallas, Texas, March, 1999.

[14] Sheen, J.H. A new look at supratip deformity. *Ann Plast Surg.* 1979;3(6):498-504.

[15] Brody, H.J. The use of hyaluronidase in the treatment of granulomatous hyaluronic acid reactions or unwanted hyalronic acid misplacement. *Dermatol Surg.* 2005;31(8 Pt 1):893-897.

[16] Hirsch R.J. Correcting superficially placed of Hyaluronic Acid. *Skin Aging.* 2007;15 (1):36-38.

Chapter 12

Auxiliary Procedures in the Nasal Skin

Guillermo Blugerman, Diego Schavelzon, Gabriel Wexler and Roberto Schale

Additional information is available at the end of the chapter

http://dx.doi.org/10.5772/62067

Abstract

Dermabrasion: This is a procedure that removes epidermis and superficial dermis in order to stimulate neo formation of collagen, elastic fibers, and vessels. **Radiofrequency:** The equipment can be regulated in ablative or nonablative (heat in dermis results in collagen fibers contraction) mode. The main effect is contraction and remodeling of collagen fibers. **Chemical peels:** Most used products are: retinoic acid, alpha hydroxy acids, trichloroacetic acid, phenol, and resorcinol. Superficial and mid peels are indicated in pigmented lesions and fine wrinkles. Deep wrinkles need a deep peel. **External nasal lifting:** As we age, flaccidity and solar damage in nasal skin turns the tip downward, and its classical correction (rhinoplasty) deepens the nasal dorsum wrinkles. Incisions and skin resection is planned in the nasoglabellar area. **Subnasal lifting:** An open nasolabial angle creates disequilibrium between the lip and nose in the central face. A buffalo horn like resection in the implantation of the nasal ala in the lip solves this angle, restoring the loss balance. **Treatment of vascular lesion with luminic energy:** Here we present our experience with nasal vascular lesions in the last 15 years. **Treatment of nasal vascular lesions through thermocoagulation with radiofrequency:** This technique is indicated in vascular lesions smaller than 3 mm of diameter, and punctiform lesions as rubi nevus and telangiectasias. **Hair removal with LASER or IPL:** The hairs anagen period of the nasal tip and vestibule gets longer as people age, turning hair to be unaesthetic.

Keywords: Chemical peels, dermabrasion, external nasal lifting, gravitational wrinkles, IPL in nasal area, LASER in nasal area, minimal invasive nasal procedure, nasal aesthetics, nasal aging, nasal dressings, nasal hair removal, nasal tip ptosis, nasal vascular lesions, nasal wrinkles, nasolabial proportions, nonablative radiofrequency, phenol peel, radiofrequency in nasal area, selective photothermolysis, subnasal lifting

1. Introduction

With aging, the nasal skin suffers the same changes as the rest of the face skin. The fact that it is medial and projected over the frontal plane makes it more vulnerable to sun radiation, having a greater risk of photoaging, preneoplastic and neoplastic lesions. As years go by, skin loses collagen fibers, elastic fibers, and subcutaneous tissue, losing volume and support. In this chapter, minimal invasive procedures for the solution of nasal skin aesthetic issues will be presented.

Caucasian thin skin tends to develop wrinkles earlier, while thicker skins develop them later. Women's skin is thinner and that is why it looks older than in a man of the same age. Smoking and sun exposure are main factors that contribute to the early development of wrinkles and sulcus. The use of heavy glasses over a long period of time can lead to skin sliding off the nasal bridge, creating wrinkles over the lateral wall of the nasal pyramid. In some cases, the material of glasses has generated chronic dermatitis.

Basically there are two types of wrinkles:

1. Expression wrinkles

2. Gravitational wrinkles

Expression wrinkles originate in mimic muscles activity, especially those superficial ones with insertions in skin around lip and eyes. The sphincter muscles such as the orbicularis oculi and orbicularis oris have mainly skin insertions and have a major function in expressing anger, worry, concentration, and other moods.

Gravity forces in any part of the face form the gravitational lines. As time passes, skin gets loose, falling over the forehead, brows, lids, nose, cheek, and neck. There is an important individual variation during this process. In the presence of atrophied skin, the aging process is faster.

As a general rule, expression wrinkles can be treated through external softening procedures or BOTOX®, and gravitational wrinkles with suspension procedures, fillers, or external lifting. There is a great amount of fillers: autologous or heterologous, absorbable or permanent. To stimulate the production of collagen, elastic fibers, and vessels, the superficial excision of epidermis and dermis can be used, creating a controlled lesion, that when healed leaves a more juvenile skin. This can be done through mechanical, chemical, physical, or electrical methods.

2. Mechanical methods: Dermabrasion

Dermabrasion is a very well-known technique [1] that was initially used for the treatment of unaesthetic scars (accidents, surgery, acne) and dysplastic lesions [2]. This procedure can be done with electrical instruments with abrasive tips of diamond or steel that spin at high speeds (Fig. 2) or water sandpaper previously sterilized (Fig. 1).

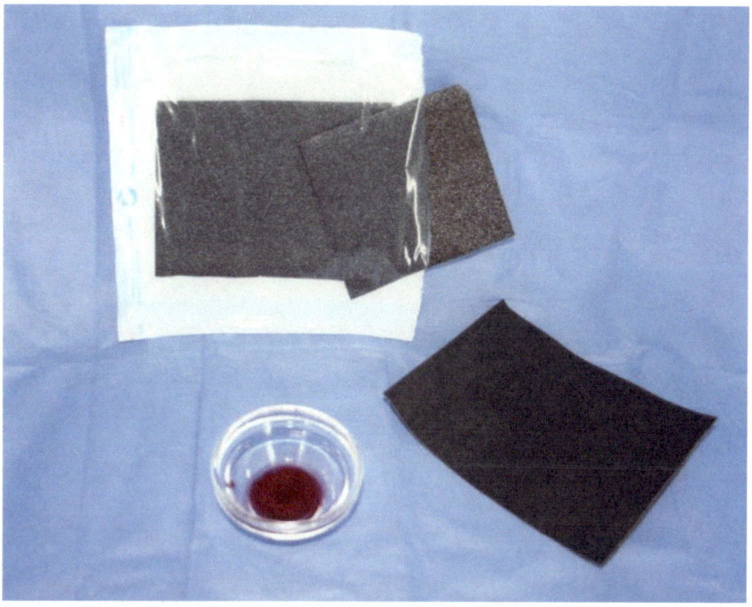

Figure 1. Materials employed in manual dermabration (left).

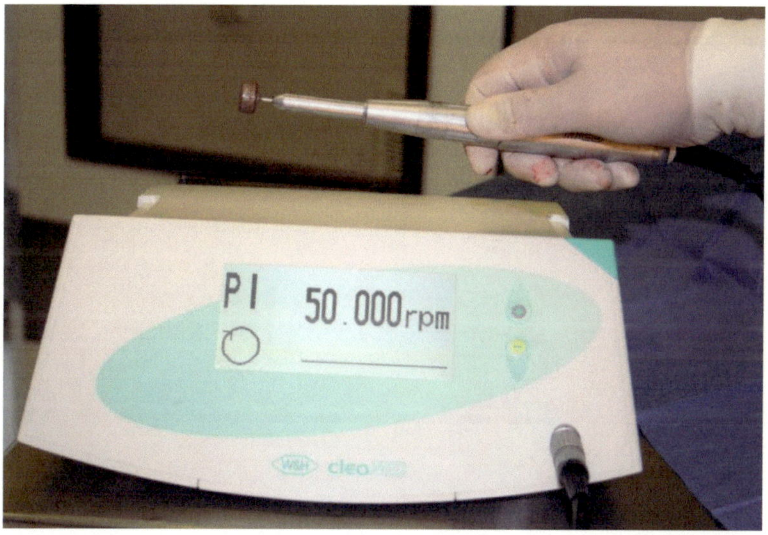

Figure 2. Equipment for high-speed dermabrasion (right).

The results of dermabrasion are very gratifying and comparable to chemical or LASER abrasion (Fig. 3). It is important not be aggressive if inexperienced because deep abrasion leave unaesthetic scars. Most frequent complication is wound infection with bacteria or herpes, with which the wound deepens and permanent scars appear.

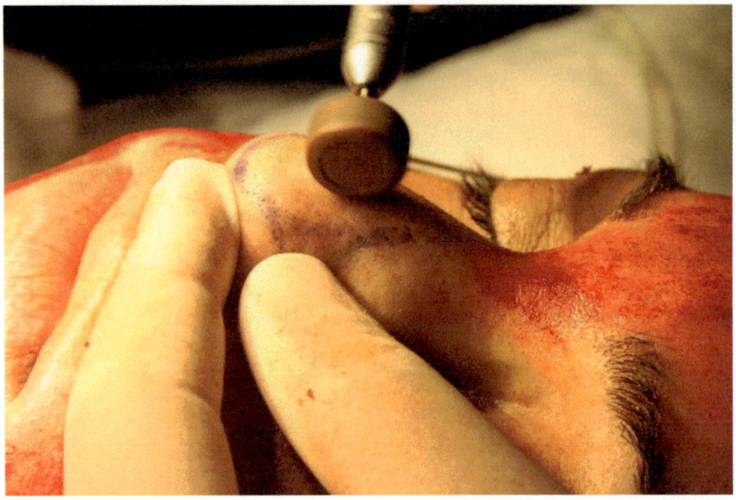

Figure 3. Dermabrasion with diamond tip.

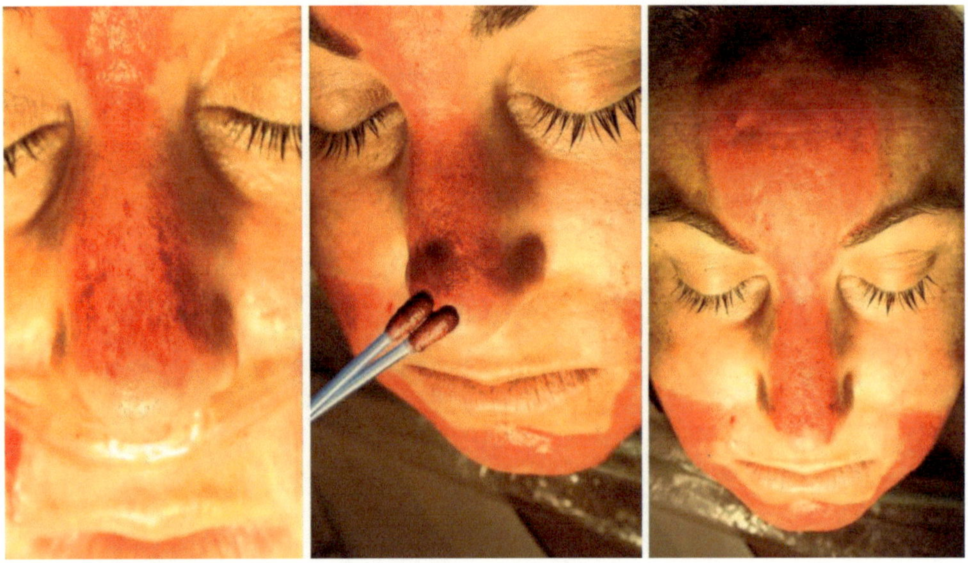

Figure 4. Blood bed and hemostasis after silver nitrate action.

In most patients, after dermabrasion we apply silver nitrate 10% over the blood bed. As a complement to the treatment, biologic dressings can be used as plasma rich in platelets (PRP), to avoid fluid loss and accelerate the healing process[3] (Figs. 4 and 5).

The procedure can be repeated after four to six months. This is the elective treatment in initial rhinophyma.

http://dx.doi.org/10.5772/62067

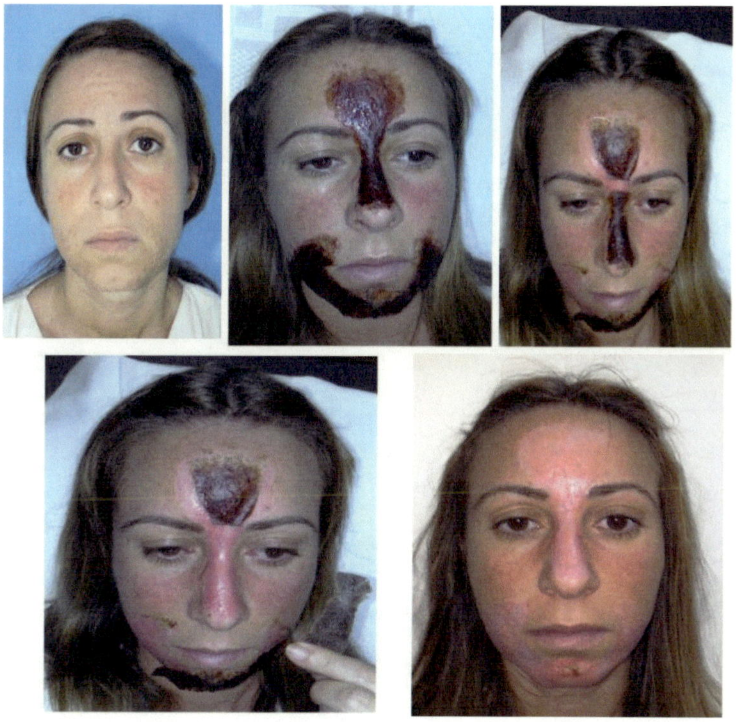

Figure 5. Preoperative, and process until the elimination of crusts left by silver nitrate.

3. Electric methods: Radiofrequency

For treatment with radiosurgery, an electronic transistorized device that produces radiofrequency waves is used [4]. This can be regulated to produce an ablative or nonablative treatment (a selective heating of the deep dermis promoting collagen fibers contraction). For the ablative treatment, we use a Surgitron 4.0 MHz of Ellman equipment with special needles and hand piece that adapt to the defect we need to correct. For the nonablative treatment, we use a Radiage hand piece, allowing us to stretch the skin without surgery (Fig. 6).

The most used radiofrequency nonablative treatment is done with Thermage equipment that produces monopolar capacitive radiofrequency. This system produces:

- Collagen fibers' immediate contraction
- Long-term collagen remodeling
- Controlled volumetric heating of tissue
- Simultaneous hand piece cooling, which protects epidermis
- Control of the heating deepness in dermis
- Possibility of normal life after the procedure

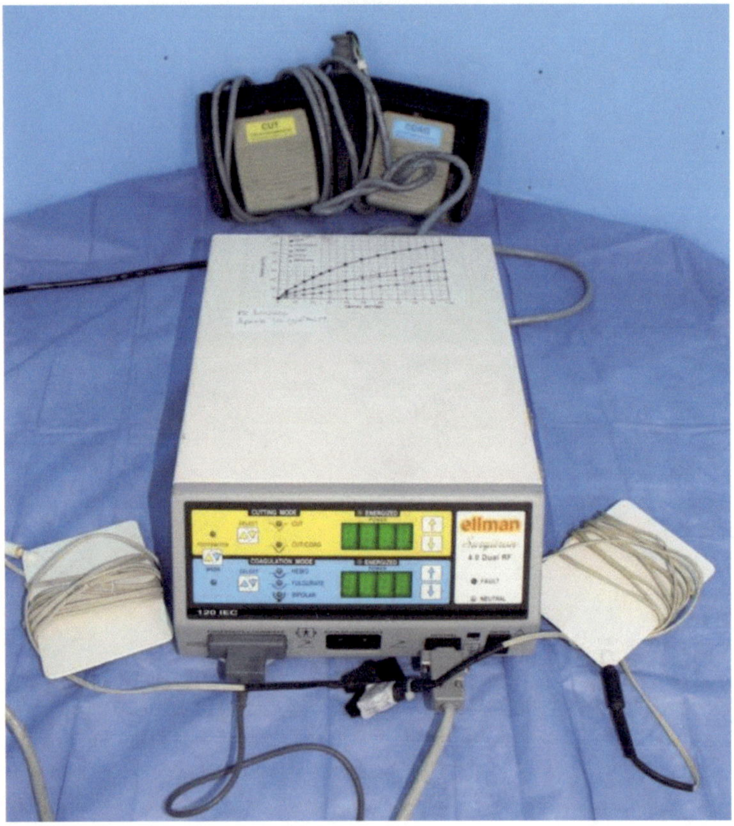

Figure 6. Ellman radiofrequency equipment.

The size and characteristics of the hand piece make its use in the nasal area difficult but using in the neighboring skin, a tightening effect is obtained in the nose.

Another equipment with which we have a positive experience is Accent of Alma Lasers that allows monopolar and bipolar modes, and has hand piece more adequate for the nose.

4. Chemical methods: Chemical peel

There are many ways to stimulate skin regeneration with acids. Taking into account the deepness of the lesions we need to treat, we choose different products to obtain a superficial, mid, or deep peel. Most used products are:

- Retinoic Acid, synthetic derived of vitamin A
- Alpha hydroxy acids, found in milk, fruits, and sugar (glycolic acid)
- Trichloroacetic acid (TCA)
- Phenol, in different concentrations

http://dx.doi.org/10.5772/62067

- Resorcinol

Superficial and mid peels are useful for treating pigmented lesions and fine wrinkles of the nasal dorsum and tip, but in the presence of deep wrinkles a deep peel is needed.

Baker-Gordon [5] formula with phenol has been the most popular deep peel in the world, but the solution instability has the risk of provoking vicious scars. That is why we prefer a commercial formula known as Exoderm [6]. This formula, created by Yoram Fintsi [7] is a modification of the Baker formula with a neutralization system. In this way, it does not transgress the basal membrane of the skin, having lesser chances of heart or kidney toxicity (Fig. 7). The formula is composed of:

- 1 ml. of liquid phenol 91%
- 1 ml. of crystal phenol 99.5%
- 2 qt. of croton oil
- 10 qt. of hexachlorophene
- 0.3 ml. of resorcinol
- 0.3 ml. of salicylic acid
- 0.5 ml. of stilled water
- 0.5 ml. of a mixture of olive oil, glycerin, ethanol, and sesame oil
- 10 ml. of hydroxymethyl aminomethane as buffer

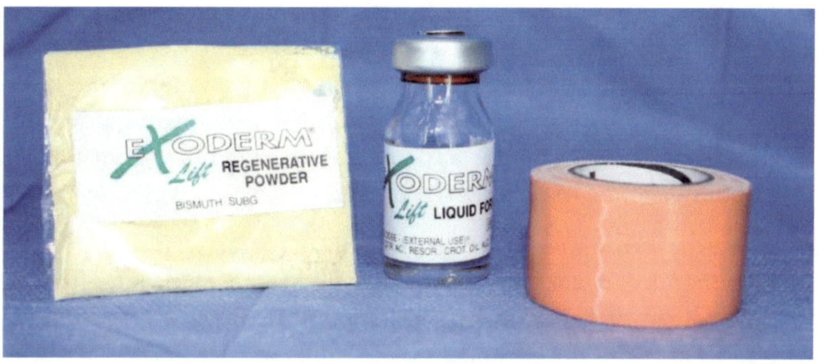

Figure 7. Commercial presentation of exoderm.

The principal indications are:

- Photoaging wrinkles
- Frown lines
- Acne scars
- Scars

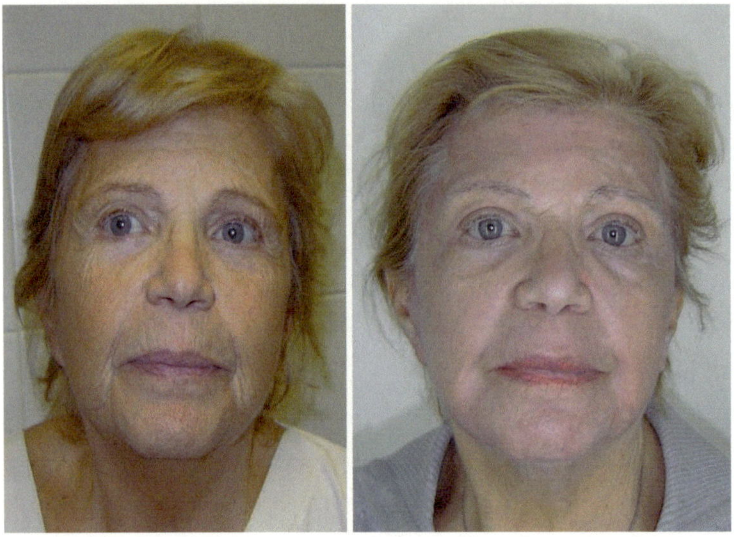

Figure 8. Pre- and postexoderm treatment.

- Pigmented lesions and keratoacanthoma
- Rhinophyma

It is fundamental to clean the skin with acetone before applying phenol to remove the skin's sebaceous content. Sedation is recommended to avoid the burning sensation. When treating the frown, nasal dorsum or tip, we must include the entire aesthetic unit. Usually, we apply the product and wait for the frosting effect, which indicates epidermal proteins denaturing. Then we evaluate if more product is needed in the entire area or just deeper lesions. The treated area can be left open in contact with air or with an occlusive bandage. If the last is done, it has to be removed the next day. After this, we use a bismuth-based healing powder, which forms a green crust that adheres to the area for approximately seven days. On day six, the patient must start using liquid vaseline to remove the crusts.

If the indication was appropriate and the procedure correctly done, positive results are expected (Fig 8). Erythema can last for eight weeks and in white skins or atrophied skins even longer. Labial herpes, heart arrhythmia, and kidney failure are absolute contraindications for this procedure. The most frequent complications are milia (a very marked line between treated and untreated skin), hyperpigmentation, hypopigmentation, and labial herpes.

5. External nasal lifting

When the skin quality, laxity, or nasal deformity cannot be corrected with the exposed methods, a surgical external nasal lifting is needed. Aging in the face affects each and every aesthetic area [8]. The central situation of the nose in the facial frame and its importance in the facial profile make it a subject of frequent consultation in patients seeking rejuvenation.

In the nose, skin alterations caused by the lack of elasticity, excessive looseness, and solar damage, causes an increase in the length of the cutaneous coverage resulting in tip ptosis. These patients, generally over their seventies, have an inelastic skin with horizontal wrinkles in the nasal bridge and lateral walls. By placing with our fingers the tip in the right position wrinkles deepen and increase significantly. In these cases, suspension techniques or fillers are useless to solve the problem. For this reduced amount of patients, in which the noninvasive procedures have poor results, we recommend the external nasal lifting, using techniques previously described for reconstructive procedures [9].

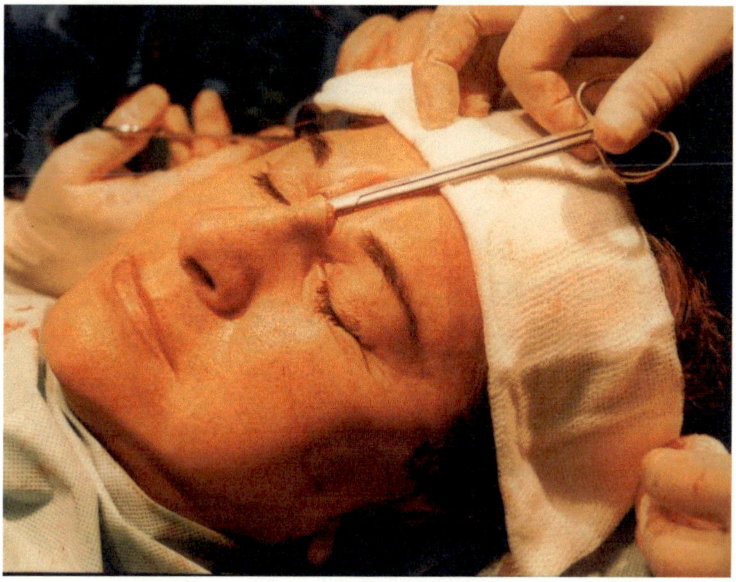

Figure 9. Picture of external nasal lifting surgical procedure.

5.1. Patient selection

The ideal candidates for this procedure are those with nasal tip ptosis caused by excessive skin looseness. These patients have usually important photoaging and are in their sixties or seventies.

5.2. Procedure

The main objective is to produce a shortening of the nasal length by resecting a block of skin over the nasal SMAS [10]. First, the skin to be removed is marked in ellipsoidal or inverted U form in the nasal bridge dorsum at the level of the medial canthus. Local infiltration is done with 1% Lidocaine with 1:100000 adrenalin in the nasal dorsum and the depressor septi nasi. The marked skin is resected respecting the SMAS plane [11]. After that we elevate a SMAS flap with inferior pedicle and we dissect below it until reaching the supratip area (Fig. 9). The SMAS flap is fixed to the periosteum of the nasofrontal joint with Nylon 5-0. Hemostasis is done.

Closure is done deep with separated stitches of Monocryl 4-0 and superficial with a continuous intracuticular suture with Monocryl 4-0. Finally, to reduce the risk of relapse, a myotomy of the depressor septi nasi is done through a small incision in the nasal vestibule or through an intraoral approach [12, 13].

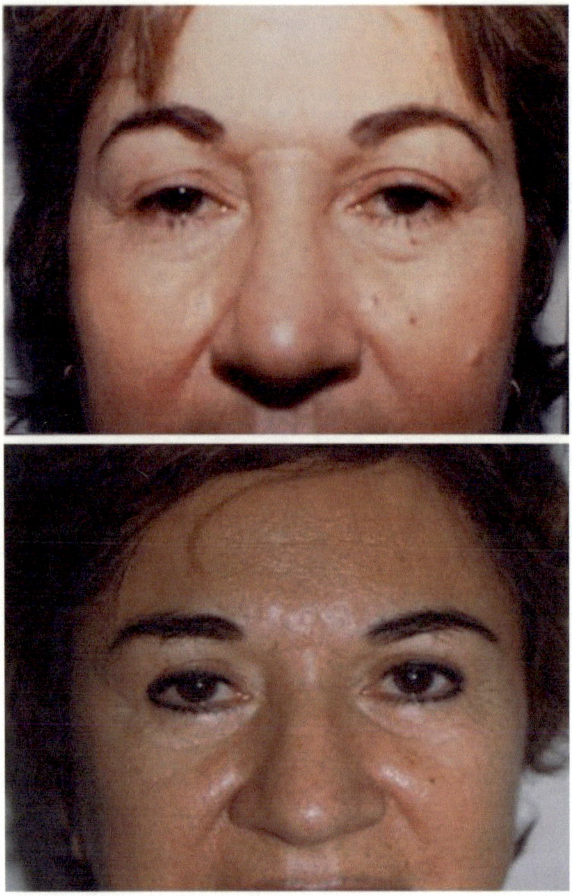

Figure 10. Before and after (8 years) external nasal lifting through previous scar. Frontal view.

We use occlusive bandage with micropore tape and thermomoldable plastic.

In general, the scar is acceptable from the aesthetic point of view and patients have a high degree of satisfaction with the procedure.

5.3. Conclusions

Nasal external lifting is a minimal invasive procedure, easy and fast to execute, without major complications. The combination with other facial rejuvenation surgical procedures does not increase significantly the surgical times (Figs. 10 and 11).

http://dx.doi.org/10.5772/62067

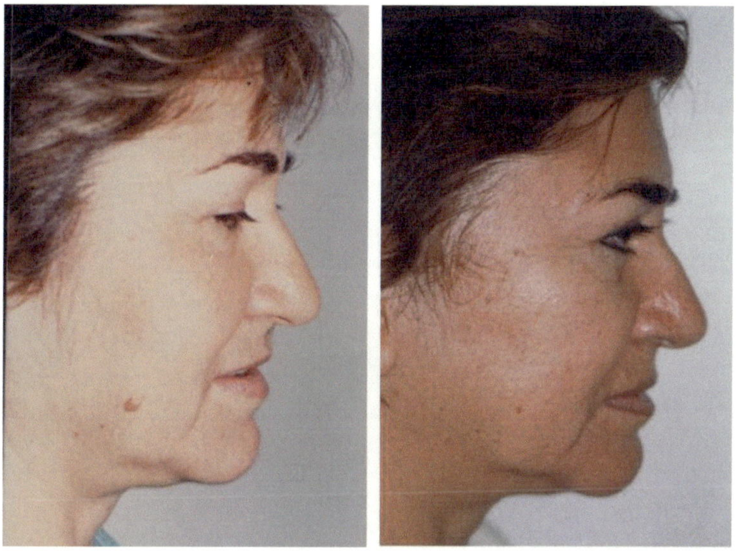

Figure 11. Before and after (8 years) external nasal lifting through previous scar. Lateral view.

6. Subnasal lifting

A over-open nasolabial angle creates disharmony between the nose and the lip, generating an unaesthetic appearance of facial features. For patients with this problem we use the subnasal lifting technique, a simple, minimal invasive procedure and one of rapid recovery. It can be done under local anesthesia, reducing the nasolabial angle (treating the depressor septi nasi), shortening the upper lip, and the vermilion is everted. A great number of men request for this surgery.

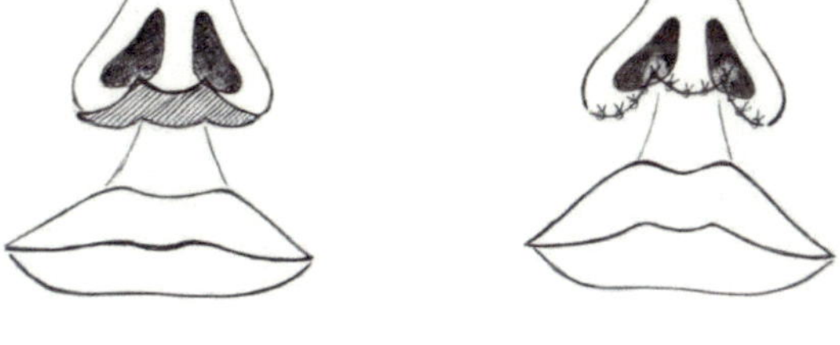

Figure 12. Buffalo horn design for skin resection.

Marking is in the form of a buffalo horn and it must be kept inside the external limit of implantation of the nasal ala to avoid visible scars (Fig. 12). Local anesthesia is done through infiltration with 1% lidocaine with adrenalin 1:100000. The resection is done following the markings, as in Fig. 13. Skin and subcutaneous tissue are resected, taking care, mainly in men, not to leave follicular units of the mustache to avoid future cystic lesions. The depressor septi nasi is treated under direct vision according to their strength, by complete or partial resection. Hemostasis is done. Skin is closed with deep and superficial stitches of Monocryl 5/0. Micropore tape is applied. Even when this technique acts mostly in the upper lip, the effect is also seen in the nose, creating a new nasolabial balance (Figs. 13 and 14).

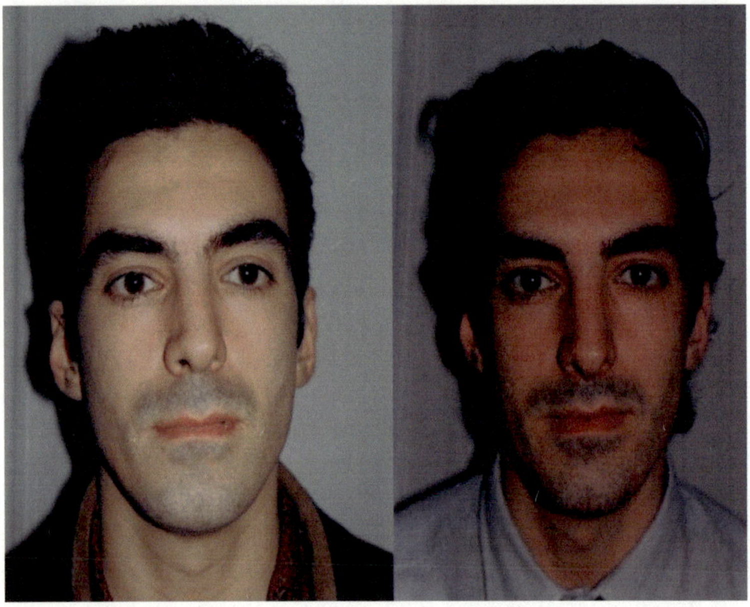

Figure 13. Before and after subnasal lifting. Frontal view.

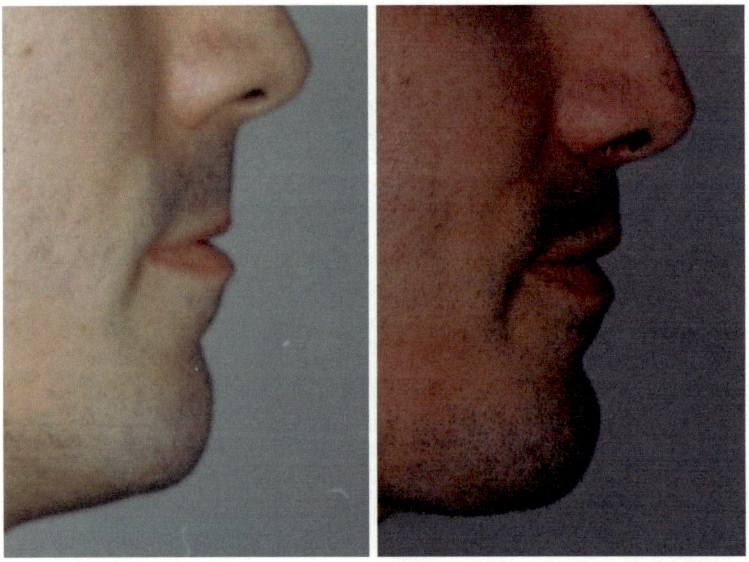

Figure 14. Before and after subnasal lifting. Observe the nasolabial angle.

http://dx.doi.org/10.5772/62067

7. Treatment of nasal vascular lesions with luminous energy

7.1. Introduction

Nasal vascular lesions are a common cause of consultation in a plastic surgery clinic. For their study, a complete clinical history is important to make the correct diagnosis and, subsequently, the correct treatment. The population that requests the removal of these lesions is growing, so we must select the best method available to minimize side effects. Nowadays, the most used methods for the treatment of these lesions are radiofrequency and luminous energy.

Vascular lesions are classified into:

- Congenital:
  - Hemangioma
  - Venous malformations
  - Port wine stains or nevus flammeus
  - Lymphangiomas
- Acquired:
  - Telangiectasias
  - Venous lakes
  - Poikiloderma
  - Cherry angiomas
  - Pyogenic granuloma
  - Rubi nevus
  - Kaposi sarcoma
  - Unspecified erythema
  - Rosacea

In general, congenital lesions have origin in vascular endothelium, arterial, venous, capillary, or lymphatic. Most frequent locations are face, neck, and extremities, but it can be located in any part of the body. They are noticed at birth or in the first weeks of life and suffer involution during childhood.

Acquired lesions are vascular dilatations, usually venous, frequently localized in face and lower extremities. There are important factors that predispose to nasal vascular lesions:

- Genetically predisposed
- Solar chronic damage
- Trauma

- Chronic treatments with steroids
- Pregnancy
- Infections
- Alcohol
- Estrogen supplements
- Rosacea

Different equipments are used according to the origin, nature, location, size, and depth of the lesion. It is important to know the working principles of these equipments in order to take the best advantage possible of them.

7.2. Luminous emission physical principles: History

Two centuries ago, only luminous emission was known. Physicists such as Newton were the first to recognize the wavy characteristic of light. Years later, they discovered that different colors corresponded to different wavelengths. In 1903, N.R. Finsen was awarded the Nobel Prize for the treatment of vulgar lupus with ultraviolet light, initiating a new field in medicine: Photomedicine. The work published by Einstein in 1917 about the controlled management of light waves was the fundamental knowledge for working with LASERS. It was not until 1933 with the discovery of optical fiber that scientists started working in microwave amplification. In 1951, this technique was patented by Fabrikant, a Russian physicist, and the year after the first equipment was built called MASER (microwave amplification by stimulated emission of radiation). In 1958, Schawlow and Townes [14] published their work in microwave amplification by stimulated emission of radiation bringing two new concepts: monochromatic light and coherent light. In 1960 [15], the first Ruby LASER was installed in the Cincinnati University. The first medical use of LASER was in ophthalmology. From there it had an exponential growth, reaching almost every field in medicine, with a great variety of equipments with different wavelength, frequency, and energy.

7.3. Physical aspects of light and LASER radiation

The transportation of energy in the form of particles generates waves with an electrical component and a magnetic one, resulting in electromagnetic radiation [16]. As these particles vary in their energy load, they have different wave length and frequency, thus completing the electromagnetic spectrum. Light is not more than electromagnetic radiation, transmitted by particles called photons, in the visible emission spectrum that has a wavelength between 300 and 700 nm.

The luminous system includes radiation with a wavelength between 200 and 1000000 nm, from ultraviolet to infrared. Most part of the radiation comes from the sun. So, radiation can be either natural (solar radiation) or artificial (LASERS and lamps). Both have emission in ultraviolet, visible, and infrared spectrum. The emission process can be coherent (LASER) or not coherent (solar light, lamps, LED).

7.4. LASER radiation

The word LASER [17] is an acronym of light amplification by stimulated emission of radiation. The characteristics of this light emission are: coherence, monochrome, directionality, intensity, and polarization. Basically, a LASER is composed by an energy source, an active medium whose molecules are exited (solid, liquid, or gas), and an amplifying system. The LASER is named after its active medium:

- Gas: CO2, argon, He-Ne
- Solid: Er.YAG, Nd. YAG
- Liquid: colorants
- Semiconductors: diode

Reflecting surfaces, as mirrors, which have a multiplicative effect and direct photons, composes the amplifying system.

7.5. Effects of light emission in tissue

According to Grothus-Drayer law, the tissues are affected when they absorb the light, transforming it into thermal and biochemical energy. There is a long list of published investigations about the interaction between light and tissues. From the optical point of view, tissues are heterogeneous, so five effects can occur when an electromagnetic light hits them:

- Reflection
- Refraction
- Transmission
- Dispersion
- Absorption

There is a great variation in medical application of LASERs because many different structures can be aimed with different equipments. There are some mathematical models that try to predict the light distribution among tissues. One of these is the Kubelka-Munk model, which provides information regarding the percentage of absorbed energy in different depth of tissue, according to tissue composition, attenuation coefficient, and absorption and dispersion phenomenon. These measurements and parameters are the fundamentals of selective photothermolysis and absorption of cellular photoreceptors.

7.6. Selective photothermolysis

In 1983, Anderson and Parish [18] discovered the light selective destruction of a structure known as chromophore or target, with minimal effects in neighboring tissue. This is based on the Thermal Relaxation Time, that is, the time necessary to reduce by 50% the maximum temperature obtained in the destruction of the structure. The effects will depend on the interaction of the following factors:

- Wavelength
- Exposition time
- Fluency (or energy density)

This mechanism is the foundation for the treatment of different lesions: pigmented, vascular, tattoos, tissue renovation, cutaneous remodeling, and hair removal. Through specific chromophores, as melanin and oxihemoglobin, light is absorbed provoking radical changes in tissue. The luminous effects can be classified in four groups:

- Electromechanic or photoacoustic: photodisruption
- Photoablation, mainly used in ophthalmology
- Thermal, vaporization, and coagulation, most known and used
- Not thermal

Not all LASERs can produce these effects, and some noncoherent light sources, such as intense pulsed light (IPL), can produce some. Up to here, we have resumed the common characteristics of light emission equipments, coherent and noncoherent. Also the physics behind the LASER has been exposed in order to know which equipment to use according to the lesion structure that is being treated. In our practice, we have these equipments since 1998; in this chapter, we will share our experience in the treatment of nasal vascular lesions with:

- Deka Smartepil Nd YAG 1064nm
- Polaris Syneron Diodo 780–980 nm combined with radiofrequency
- Fotona XP Max Nd YAG 1064nm

The nasal vascular lesions that we have treated in the last 15 years include: plane angioma (cavernous, lobular, senile, serpinginous), facial telangiectasias, erythema, rosacea, and rubi nevus. A detailed clinical history is done taking into account the following:

- Type of lesions
- Phototype
- Localization
- History of the lesions
- Personal history
- Family history
- Medication
- Previous treatments
- Type of skin
- Pictures of the lesions

- Extended explanation of possible complications of the treatment
- Informed Consent

7.7. Technique

The preparation for the treatment is common for any equipment. Pictures of the area are taken. The equipment is programmed with the correct parameters to treat a specific lesion. Both, the patient and the doctor, must wear protective glasses.

For the treatment of nasal telangiectasia small spot LASERs are preferred; with IPL it is harder to adapt the hand piece to the treatment. It is important to check after the first shot the response in the vascular walls and skin covering the vessel. According to that response, parameters are adjusted in order to obtain the best result with least collateral damage. Cooling the skin is not recommended because it causes vasoconstriction, removing oxihemoglobin (the aimed chromophore) from vessels (Fig. 15). This is a very extensive mistake, and we think it is because doctors or technicians use the same methodology as for other applications (hair removal, facial rejuvenation, tattoo removal) with fixed chromophores (melanin, ink) in which cooling is very effective in reducing pain and side effects. Once finished with the treatment, an immediate effect is observed; this percentage of improvement is written down in the clinical history, together with the equipment used and the parameters.

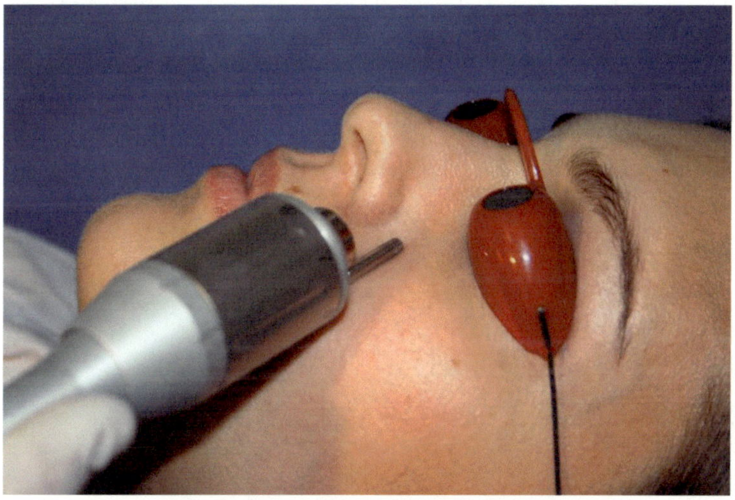

Figure 15. Nd:YAG LASER in nasal telangiectasia.

7.8. Parameters

According to the device equipments characteristics and the treatment to perform, they are used with different forms of energy, fluency, and pulse duration. The equipments we will discuss are the ones we have been using in the last 15 years, and the parameters are useful just for reference since each patient has a different requirement. The following data are for nasal telangiectasias. It is important to know, as treatment background, that limits of oxyhemoglobin absorption are between 418 and 577 nm, with a pulse duration of 10–20 ms.

7.8.1. Deka Smartepil II

With this equipment, there is a great variety of spots, we generally use a 2 mm one, wavelength of 1064 nm, maximum energy of 150 J/cm^2, pulse duration of 16 mseg, with time between pulses up to 300 mseg. Up to 7 mm spots can be used that allow higher fluency up to 200 J/cm^2, but in this area of the face we do not recommend it.

7.8.2. Polaris Syneron ELOS

This is the only equipment, in our practice, that allows luminous energy treatment simultaneously with radiofrequency. Its power source is a diode, which produces a wavelength between 780 and 980 nm. Luminous energy can be used between 10 and 140 J/cm^2, and radiofrequency between 10 and 100 J/cm^2 with a spot of 5 x 5 mm.

7.8.3. Fotona XP II

This is an Nd-Yag LASER, with a wavelength of 1064 nm, maximum energy of 120 J/cm^2, pulse duration between 5 and 200 mseg, and a 20 mm spot. This is the same equipment as for endolaser treatment of varicose veins (Fig. 16).

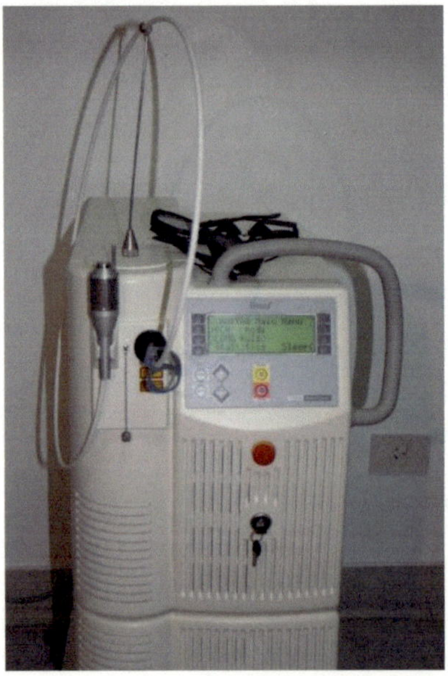

Figure 16. LASER FOTONA XP.

After the treatment is finished, cooling of the skin is done with ice or gel packs for a few minutes.

Apart from the mentioned equipments, there are others with the ability to produce selective photothermolysis:

LASER type	Wavelength in nm
Argon	488–514
Copper vapor	578
Krypton	568
KTP	532

7.9. Posttreatment indications

Indications and precautions are common for most equipments. Erythema can be experienced in the first hours and cooling devices usually solve it. The treated area should not be exposed to sun light, and tanning beds are forbidden for ten days after the treatment. Solar protection factor (SPF) over 40 should be used. If the patient has not experienced any complications, the treatment is repeated after day 21 until erasing of the lesion.

7.10. Side effects and complications

Complications of this treatment almost never end in permanent sequel. The most frequent side effect is erythema, which usually lasts between 6 and 48 hours after the treatment, disappearing spontaneously.

Vesicles of 1–3 mm can appear in the treated area; this is because vessels are very superficial, thus transmitting heat to the skin, or responding to an excess in the energy used. They usually heal spontaneously in few days. Steroid healing creams are recommended and sun exposure is forbidden.

The most serious complications are hypertrophic scars and keloids, but in the nasal area atrophic and hypopigmented scars are more frequent.

In the last years, there has been an important reduction of complications rate due to a better knowledge of this technology and of the biological response to it.

Prevention is essential: correct patient choice, avoiding tanned skins, complete knowledge of the equipment, and periodical equipment technical services. Constant training is necessary for personnel using the equipments. Following these principles, complications are reduced to a minimum, and the treatment turns safe and efficient.

Absolute contraindications for this treatment are:

- Photosensitivity
- Anticoagulation

- Low platelets level
- Convulsive syndrome triggered by light
- Treatment with photosensitive drugs
- Phototype VI of Fitzpatrick

7.11. Conclusions

The technical advances in LASER technology have made possible the treating of most skin vascular lesions. With the increase in energy density, wavelength, exposition time, the association of these parameters, and the added effect of radiofrequency, these equipments are entering every field of medicine. Constant training is needed in order to apply new technologies with a safety margin for patients.

8. Definitive hair removal with laser or IPL

The follicular units of the nasal tip have an anagen period that enlarges with age, thus growing a thicker hair as the years go by. The same occurs with hair in the nasal vestibule, which is highly unaesthetic. Changing some parameters in the mentioned equipments, melanin can be aimed as chromophore. So, based on the selective photothermolysis principle, follicular units from the nasal tip, ala, and vestibule can be eliminated. Five to six sessions with a 45–60 days interval are needed in order to obtain a permanent reduction in the number of active follicles using LASER or IPL. The patient should not be tanned during the treatment in order to avoid burns and hypopigmentation.

9. Radiofrequency thermocoagulation of nasal vascular lesions

Radiofrequency (RF) is another type of energy that has been used to alter skin connective tissue. Its use in medicine has a history of more than 70 years, but recent equipments can deliver the energy selectively to the deep dermis and subdermis. In the late 1990s, equipments were adapted for skin ablation, generating plasma at different deepness of skin. Recently, this technology was reconfigured for nonablative use in aesthetic medicine. The impact of RF on skin depends on the tissue impedance (Ohms), the RF power (Watts), the exposition time (seg), and the electrode configuration.

The radiofrequency thermocoagulation technique allows erasing vascular punctate lesions smaller than 3 mm such as Ruby nevus, cuperosis, small varicose lesions, and telangiectasia. The treatment is based on the thermal effect of a high-frequency wave that is focused in a fine needle. The varicose lesion disappears instantly, leaving a wheal that is replaced later by crusts. A disposable Teflon-coated nickel or gold needle of 0.075 mm diameter is used (Fig. 17). This reduces chances of allergic reactions, and thermal diffusion.

The treatment can be performed in a private office; it usually lasts for 15–10 min, and the posttreatment indications are similar to the ones mentioned for LASER. Topical anesthesia creams or cooling devices can be used in order to reduce pain during the procedure.

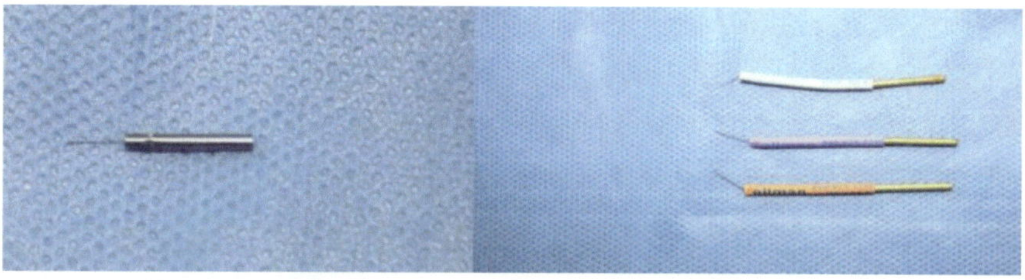

Figure 17. Needles used for radiofrequency cauterization of nasal telangiectasia.

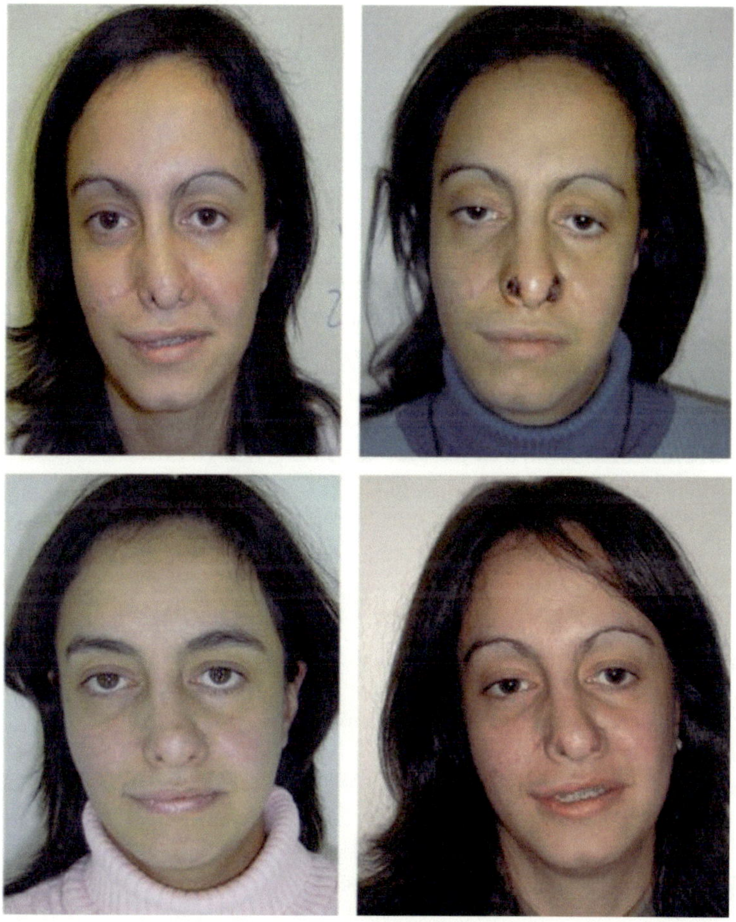

Figure 18. Before and after various auxiliary procedures for treatment of accident sequels.

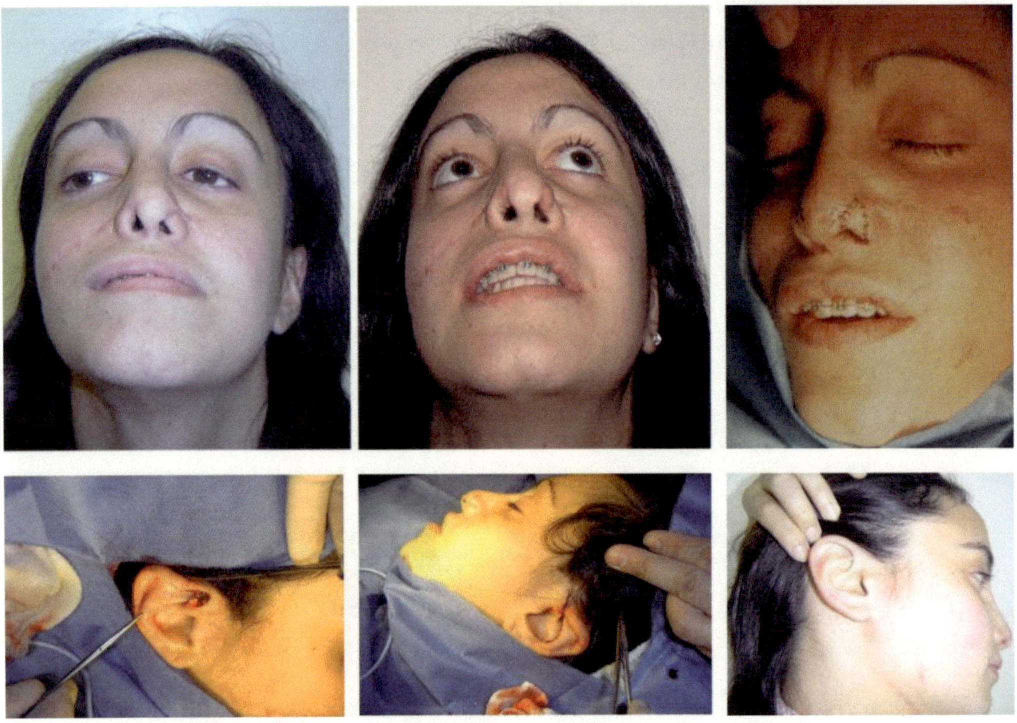

Figure 19. Nasal ala reconstruction with auricular compound graft, complemented with dermabrasion and PMMA.

Thermocoagulation is a safe technique that selectively delivers energy to the vascular lesion, preserving the epidermis. This procedure can be done in every season, in any kind of skin, is not painful, and does not require posttreatment bandages. The only drawback is that in every site treated the patient will have for some days a crust, and for some patients this is socially unacceptable. Effectiveness is seen in the first session (Figs. 18 and 19).

Author details

Guillermo Blugerman[1*], Diego Schavelzon[1], Gabriel Wexler[2] and Roberto Schale[1]

*Address all correspondence to: blugerman@centrosbys.com

1 Plastic Surgery Department of Centros ByS, Centros B&S de Excelencia en Cirugía Plástica, Argentina

2 Universidad Nacional del Nordeste, Argentina

Conflict of interest: none. Authorized consent was obtained from the patients included in the chapter.

References

[1] Petres, J., Rompel R., Robins P. *Dermabration. Dermatologic Textbook and Atlas Surgery*. Berlin, 1996. Springer. pp. 39-41.

[2] Horibe E.K. *Estética Clínica y Quirúrgica*. Rio de Janeiro, 2000. Revinter: pp. 77-83.

[3] Blugerman G. Utilización de Plasma Rico en Plaquetas como curativo de la Dermoabrasión Quirúrgica, In: *Procedimientos Esteticos Mínimamente Invasivos Coor*. Charles Yamaguchi, Sao Pablo, 2006 Editorial Santos. pp.173-182

[4] Filippo Alexandre. Radiofrecuencia, In: *Procedimientos Estéticos Mínimamente Invasivos Coor*. Charles Yamaguchi. Sao Pablo, 2006 Editorial Santos. pp. 273-274.

[5] Baker T.J. Chemical face peeling and rhydectomy. *Plast Reconstr Surg Transplant Bull*. 1962;29:199-207.

[6] Schavelzon D. Nuestra Experiencia con Exoderm en Rejuvenecimiento Facial. *Procedimientos Estéticos Mínimamente Invasivos Coor*. Charles Yamaguchi. Sao Pablo, 2006, Editorial Santos. pp. 165-172.

[7] Fintsi Y., Landau M. Exoderm: Fenol based peeling in olive and dark skinned patients. *Int J Cosm Surg Aesthet Dermatol*. 2001;3:173-178.

[8] Gonzalez-Ulloa, M. Restoration of the FACE covering by jeans of selected skin in regional aesthetic units. *Br J Plast Surg*. 1956;9(3):212-221.

[9] Jackson Ian T. *Colgajos Locales en la Reconstrucción de Cabeza y Cuello*. Barcelona, 1990, Salvat Editores. pp. 136-137.

[10] Letourneau A., Daniel R.K. The superficial musculoaponeurotic system of the nose. *Plast Reconstr Surg*. 1988;82(1):48-57.

[11] Cheffe, Luis Oscar. Metodizaçäo eclética para tratamento do lábio senil com modificaçöes táticas Anais do Simpósio Brasileiro do Contorno Facial, Sociedade Brasileira de Cirurgia Plástica. 1983. pp. 244-247.

[12] Perenack J. Lip modification procedures as an adjunct to improving smile and dental esthetics. *Atlas Oral Maxillofac Surg Clin N. Am*. 2006;14(1):51-74.

[13] Randolph Waldman S. The subnasal lift. *Facial Plast Surg Clin N Am*. 2007;15(4): 513-516.

[14] Schalow Al., Townes C.H. Infrared and optical Masers. *Phys Rev*. 1958;112:1940-1949.

[15] Maimann Th. Stimulated optical radiation in ruby. *Nature* 1960;187:493-494.

[16] Colls J. *Enfoque Conceptual de las Radiaciones Electromagnéticas*. La Paz. 1987 CDL; pp 1-5.

[17] Kubelka P. New contributions to the optics of intensity light scattering materials. Part II: Nonhomogeneous layers. *J Opts Soc Am.* 1954;44:330-335.

[18] Anderson R.R., Parish J.A. Selective photothermolysis precise microsurgery by selective absorption of pulsed radiation. Science 1983;220:524-527.

Chapter 13

Medical Rhinoplasty – Profile Correction with Resorbable Fillers

Alessio Redaelli

Additional information is available at the end of the chapter

http://dx.doi.org/10.5772/62066

Abstract

The correction of nasal profile is a typical surgical field dating back centuries. In the last decade, with the fabrication of resorbable fillers, a new technique, which is mini-invasive, has emerged. For this treatment, the study of patients is especially important. The procedure can be performed with needles or cannulas; is very simple and easy; and the results are immediate. It must become baggage of any aesthetic doctor.

Keywords: Medical rhinoplasty, rino-filler, hyaluronic acid, nasal profile, nasal bridge, Asian rhinoplasty, Far-East rhinoplasty, blunt cannula, nasal tip, Rhinion, Nasion, deep nasal bridge, nonsurgical rhinoplasty, nasal spine, beauty, symmetry, asymmetry

1. Introduction

I remember perfectly, when back in 2007, after having extensively corrected a lady for many problems of aging, something in her face seemed wrong and not beautiful. During a conversation, she mentioned that she had noticed also that her nose was getting progressively older. My patient did not have a particularly bad or hooked nose that required immediate correction. She had one of those typically European noses, with a slight plunge, with the root deeper than just the tip. The tip was typically slightly hypoprojected.

In that moment, all of a sudden it occurred to me that a small injection of resorbable filler, hyaluronic acid in this case, at the level of the nasal root might give an interesting aesthetic result, improving that "sad" nose.

I used a small portion of the gel in the syringe in my hand to get the required correction. The result was immediate and dazzling!

I gave the lady a mirror to see the result. She looked in disbelief for a few seconds and blurted out: "Doctor, it is incredible. All my life I wanted to improve my nasal profile, but I had always been afraid to meet a surgeon for this."

In fact, the result obtained on nasal profile after correction with an absorbable filler is instantly visible in contrast to that obtained with the botulinum toxin for all mimic problems.

The route was mapped out.

Thereafter, it was easy to obtain the correction also of the nasal tip, in all hypoprojected noses; Finally, the correction of the columellar line allows the nasal base to be slightly rotated to achieve the typical, satisfactory result.

Subsequently, in 2008 [1], I published a scientific article with details of the technique that is described in this chapter.

Of course, there are a lot of anatomical differences among the races of the world and nasal defects widely differ.

The aim of this chapter is to demonstrate to the readers the technique I use on typical European patients. These corrections, however, can be used in patients of all races that present with these defects. According to my experience, these defects are more frequent in Caucasian ladies and men, and hence the title of this chapter: "Profile correction for European Patients."

2. Study of patients and good indication

In my opinion, it is impossible to reduce nasal aesthetics to a standard template, but to understand exactly the best indication it is of fundamental importance to study our patients. The defects to be corrected are sometimes so minimal yet strongly visible; at other times, the defects are more significant but affect total aesthetic of the face to a lesser degree. I would like, in this section of the chapter, to quickly recall the main aesthetical angles of the nose, which are of fundamental importance and thereafter deal with the correction by filler.

The nose is an organ of central importance. It is in the center of the face and is obviously closely related to the neighboring areas and in particular to the frontal, malar-zygomatic, and chin areas.

The more important anatomical details have been discussed in the previous chapter and in other parts of this book, which the the reader, if needed, can access.

I recall here very briefly the skeletal classes by Angle, already mentioned in the previous chapter regarding the treatment of mimical patients, but much more important with regard to the treatment of nasal contouring.

I recount for readers who have opened the book at this page, that the skeletal classes by Angle, from a dental point of view, are very important from a purely aesthetic perspective, determining with accuracy the mutual expression and projection of the chin and nasal tip [1-4].

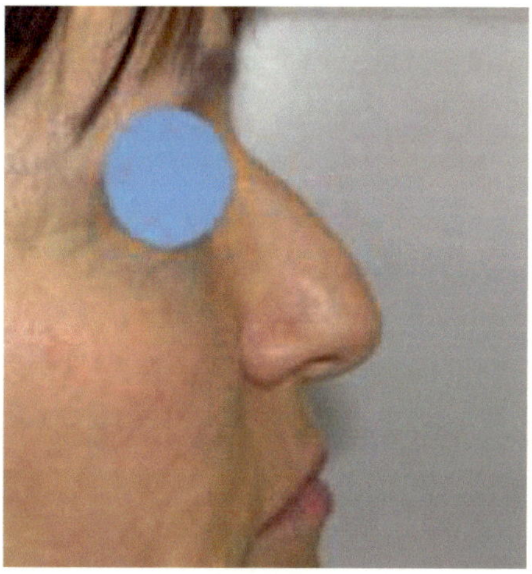

Figure 1. Please add caption

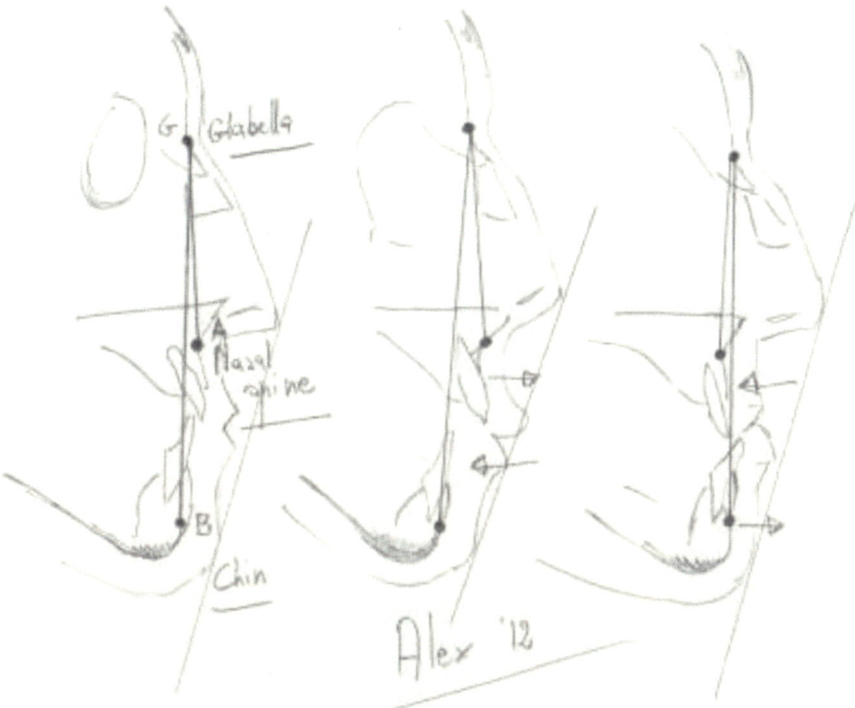

Figure 2. Angle's skeletal classes.

Edward Angle, in the past century, determined exactly what the relationships between the dental arches are, clearly observed in the lateral projection, and then described the three main models that are precisely the three skeletal classes: the first class called normal, a second class when the jaw is in a position rearward from the upper jaw, and finally a third skeletal class in which the jaw is shifted forward and the lower incisors can be on the same axis of the superior if not exactly in front of them with a typical reversed bite.

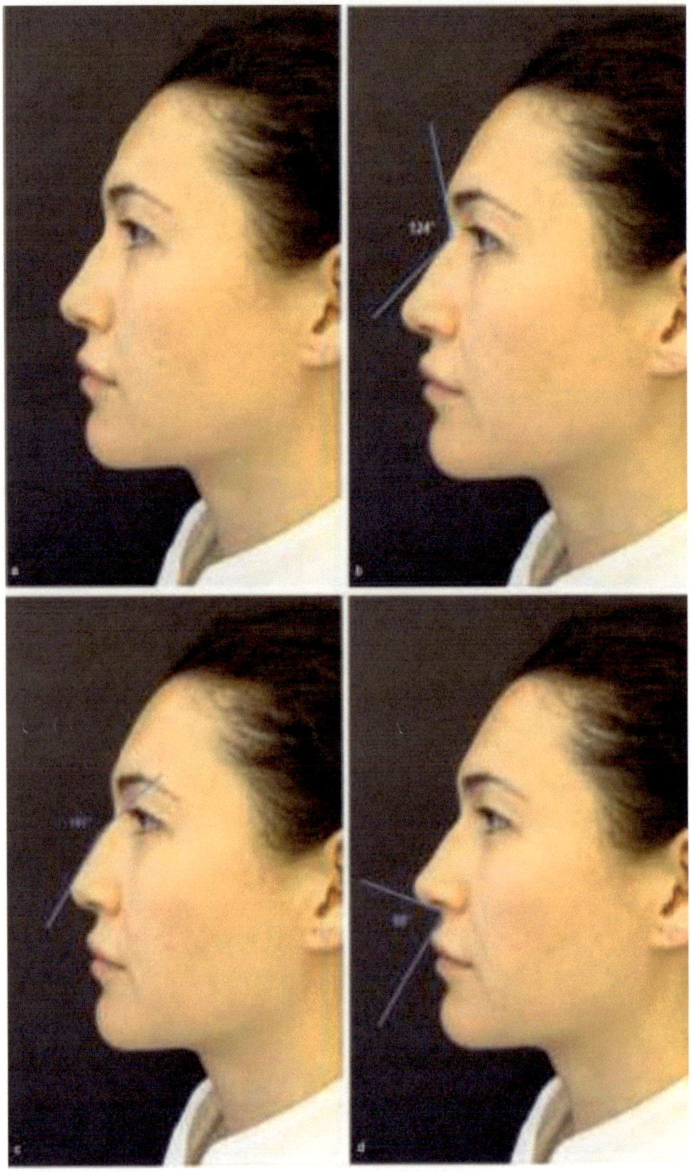

Figure 3. Main nasal angles: (a) picture of the patient in profile position; (b) naso frontal angle: normally from 130° to 145°; (c) dorsal angle: normally straight; (d) naso labial angle: normally from 90° to 110°.

It is immediately evident that in the second skeletal class, often associated with a reduced projection of the malar-zygomatic area, the nose can sometimes appear hyperprojected and bigger than it really is. As I often say in my master classes, a mountain is a mountain also because at the sides it has deep valleys!

This confirms that the nose cannot be studied in isolation, but that all facial areas in their totality are of paramount importance.

The facial angles of the nose are also of fundamental importance [1,2]. We can see them in the pictures (Figure 3).

3. Indicated fillers

Among commercial fillers, the most suitable for the correction of the nasal profile and used everyday in my surgery are those materials based on average cross-linked hyaluronic acid. It is of paramount importance that these gels are produced by pharmaceutical companies to absolute safety, with a well-known history and unequivocally perfect. I strongly advise all colleagues to avoid buying products only because they are cheap: a low price often hides a limitation in quality [2,4].

The fillers that I normally use for nasal profilometry are summarized in Table 1. I would like to emphasize that there are probably a lot of other fillers in the market that are not listed in the table, probably better than these, which I do not know of and therefore have not utilized.

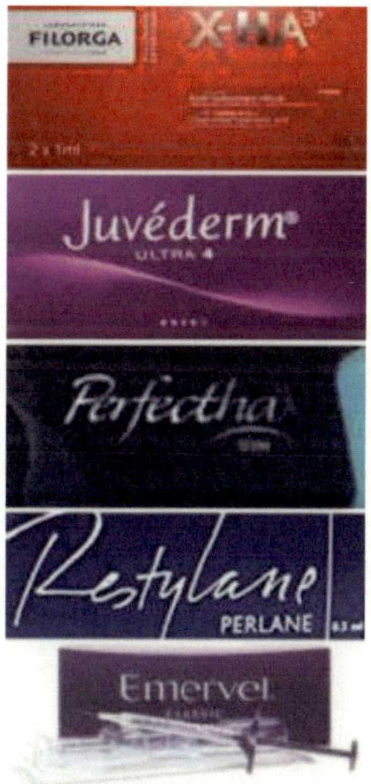

Table 1. Fillers that I normally use for nasal profilometry.

As visible in the table here above, I'm not usual to use fillers made by HA too reticulated. In my opinion, the volumetrical fillers, for nasal reshape, are not indicated. For the same reason, I do not use Calcium-hydroxyl-apatite, which is, instead, very good for volumetrical corrections.

Also all nonresorbable fillers are not used in my practice.

Fillers based on Poli-levo-lactic acid are not indicated for nasal reshaping and not used by me.

4. Correction of the nasal profile in caucasian patients with needles

The correction technique of the nasal profile in Caucasian patients with fillers foresees two techniques: with needles and cannulas.

Generally, all techniques with needles may be more dangerous due to the possibility of injecting directly into a vein or an artery. Regarding the nasal area in the strict sense, nasal sides are particularly dangerous for the presence of numerous small terminal arterioles coming from the facial artery. Particular attention must therefore be paid in the injection of this area, in particular in the subcutaneous tissue upon the triangular cartilage.

Also the area of the nasal tip can be dangerous for the possible onset of ischemia of the tip with consequent damage to the cutaneous trophism, both for matter of compression both for local injections of small terminal arterioles.

Finally, the intra-arterial injection of the columellar artery is reported with ischemia of the tissues of the nasal tip and base.

All these possible side effects have consequently introduced the use of blunt cannulas that allow us to bring down these risks to practically zero.

4.1. Correction of the nasal root

In most Caucasian patients we find the typical "Dorsal angle" over 180°.

In Fig. 5 we can see a case of a Caucasian patient during treatment. The nasal profile has the typical angle of about 190°. We use in this case a middle reticulated hyaluronic acid. The injection is made from Rhinion to Nasion. It is injected deep on the bone. It is mandatory to keep the first and second finger of the non-injecting hand closely on the sides of the nose to absolutely avoid the migration of the Hyaluronic acid on the sides of the nasal root. A migration even to the inferior eyelid is described. So great attention must be paid to this detail!

I normally use a linear retrograde technique arriving to inject 0,20,3 ml. It is better not to overcorrect. As always if the injection is not enough we can reinject. If we inject too much, it is difficult to retrace!

After the injection, a light massage to the area is useful to make uniform the implant. The result is definitely immediate (Fig. 5e).

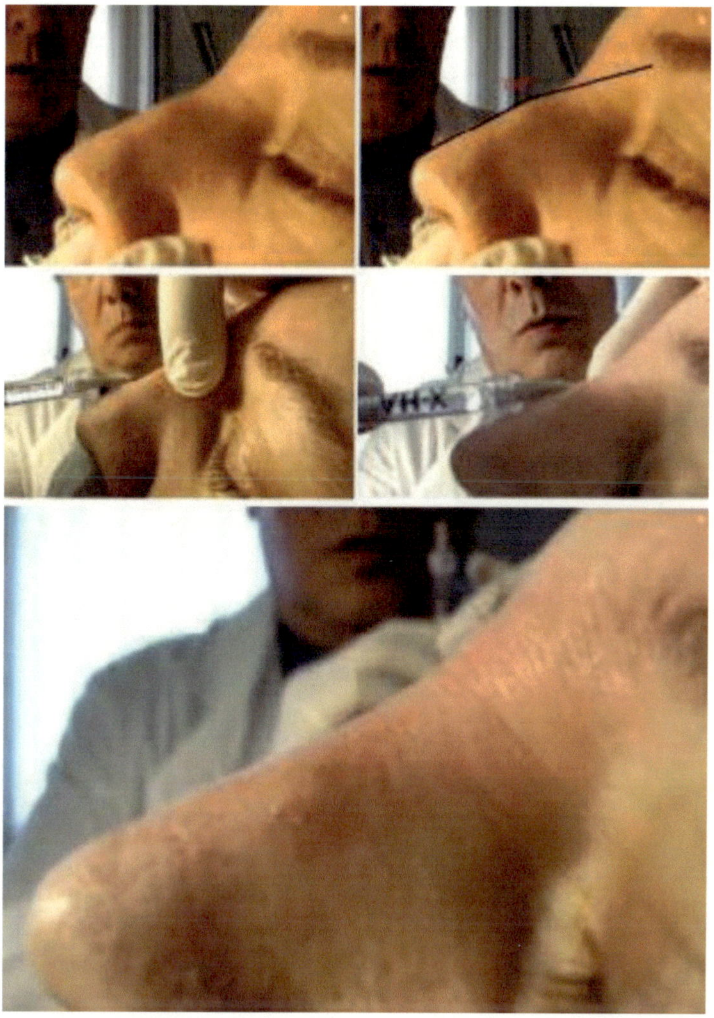

Figure 4. Correction of the nasal root.

4.2. Correction of the nasal spine

The nasolabial angle is the second angle that is sometimes reduced. This angle can be modified for mimical reasons or for a volumetrical/skeletal problem.

The correction in mimical patients can be made with BTxA (see the specific chapter).

If the problem is volumetrical, the correction can be achieved with the injection of Hyaluronic acid at the columellar area.

Normally, naso-labial angle is around 90° to 110°. The injection of nasal spine allows both an improving of the columellar line, with an opening of this angle, and also a light rotation of the nasal tip, with a better projection. In Fig. 6b, it is possible to see a not too closed nasal angle (a little bit more than 90°), but there is indication for the rotation of the nasal tip.

The injection of the nasal spine is made with a 27G x 14 mm needle (the grey one). The angle on injection can be parallel to the nasal spine–Pogonion line (Fig. 6c) in all cases of reduced angles below 85°.

If instead we need an improving of volumes, we can inject with a 45° (Fig 6d).

It is better, before injecting that a quick aspiration is made with the same injecting hand, to confirm avoiding injecting of the columellar artery.

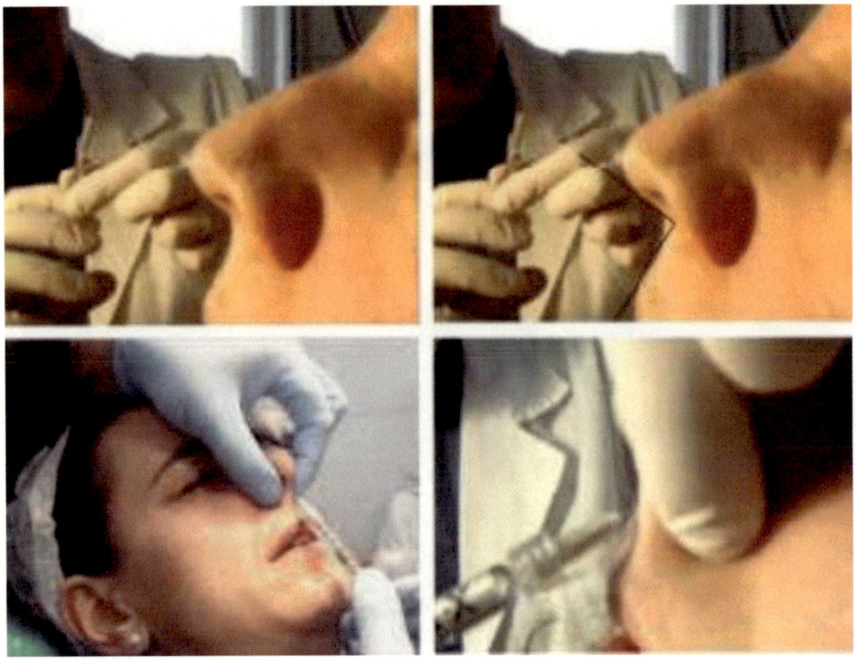

Figure 5. Injection of the nasal spine (c) and position of the contralateral fingers (d).

As visible in the figures above, the contralateral hand is helping to close the injection area and preventing loss of the product into depths where it would be not helpful to open the nasolabial angle. It is better to suggest the patient breathes with the mouth, since the nostrils will be closed with your fingers.

4.3. Correction of the nasal tip

The hypoprojected tips are the best indication.

The injection is made in the subcutaneous tissue, between the intermediate crus of the alar major cartilages. In Fig. 7b it is possible to see the exact point. The injecting doctor must decide if it is better to underline 1 or 2 tip defining points. Normally, I achieve this definition through the same entry point using a fun technique that allows us to distribute the HA gel in a perfect way.

Every nose is, of course, different from others and it is impossible give the readers a standard template.

The result is immediate and in Fig. 7d it is possible to see it in this particular patient, immediately after the procedure.

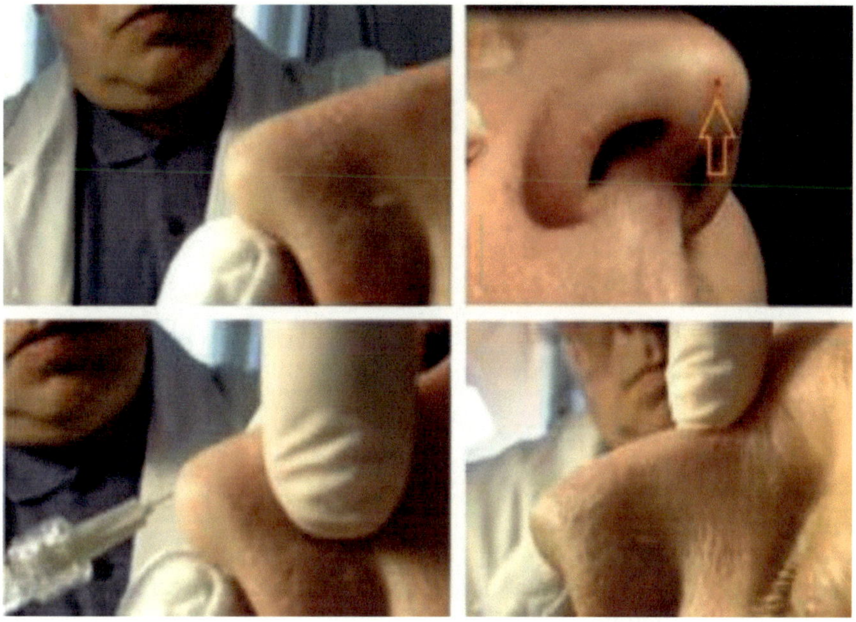

Figure 6. PLEASE ADD CAPTION

5. Correction of the nasal profile in caucasian patients with the cannula

In the last months of the 2012, I was conducting a course on Medical Rhinoplasty in Singapore for the American Academy of Aesthetic Medicine. A very kind doctor let us use his private practice for our courses. The courses on medical Rhinoplasty are very famous and followed by many doctors here in Europe and in the Far East.

After finishing my presentation, we discussed some practical casesand also Dr Kelvin Chua showed us his technique with a blunt cannula. It was surprising and really amazing the ease with which the reshaping of the nasal profile could be performed. Immediately I also understood the possibility of reducing all side effects due to injection in the vascular vessels that could be avoided with a cannula in most cases.

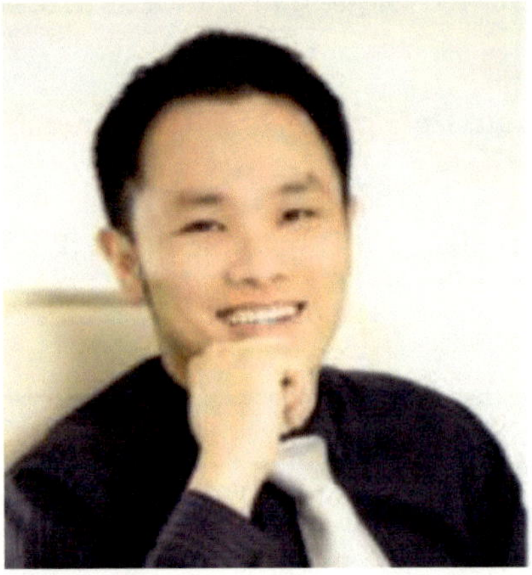

Figure 7. Dr K. Chua.

Since then I have used this new technique in a lot of cases, both for Far Eastern patients as also in many cases of European profile corrections.

In this chapter of the book by Prof. Nikolay Serdev, I would want to deeply thank this colleague for his kindness and for having opened my mind to this "Columbus's Egg" of the mini-invasive techniques on the nose.

This technique is very easy, safe, and described in the following text.

5.1. Indications

The best indication for the correction of nasal profile with the blunt cannula are the irregular profiles from the nasal tip to the root. The best cannulas to be used in this case are 25G x 50 mm. It is possible to use also 27G x 40 mm, but these are in my opinion a little bit more dangerous and also painful. Anesthesia, anyway, is not needed except for anesthetic cream at the entry point.

Patients are asked to arrive in my clinic with no makeup. The entire nasal area is thoroughly disinfected.

The cannula is inserted at the nasal tip. It is important to make the entry point at the perfect level; the entry with the cannula should be neither too superficial nor too deep.

The subcutaneous tissue is the perfect layer.

In most patients, I use a needle 23G to make the entry point at the nasal tip (Fig. 9b). The 23 G needle allows a very easy entry of the cannula, while the pain is the same as of any other thinner needle. With the preparation with the anesthetic cream, this pain is really very tolerable.

In this case I am using, as in most patients, a 25G cannula x 50 mm. The cannula is inserted gently at the entry point, and the right plain is found, where the cannula proceeds without an important pressure. The proceeding of the cannula must be easy and totally painless.

The first and second fingers of the non-injecting hand are positioned on the sides of the nose, just near the cannula to avoid spreading of the gel on the sides of the nose. This is also very useful to have a narrow nasal profile.

The cannula can arrive, however, also on the nasal sides to improve the little defects between the nasal cartilages.

Results are immediate. I suggest patients come back for a possible retouch in 15 days, since there is quite frequently a modest decrease in the result.

The result in most patients is very long-lasting, normally at least 1 year, and in many cases also 2 years.

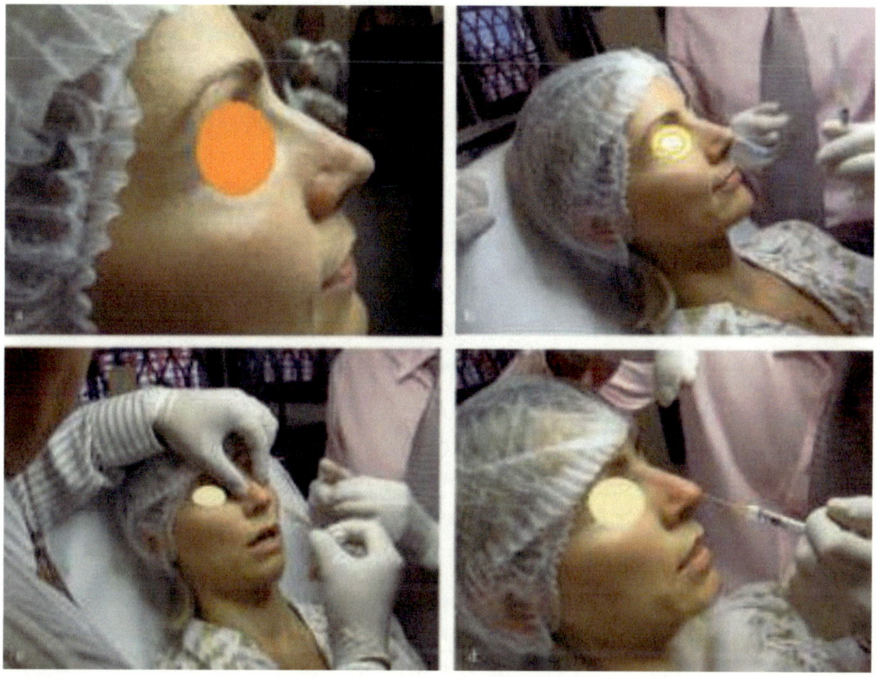

Figure 8. Please add caption

6. The profile correction for far eastern patients: the deep nasal bridge

In the previous chapter, we discussed and examined how to improve the nasal profile in Caucasian patients, especially central-European patients, both in women and in men.

I learnt of another interesting indication, and a very special one, in my many trips to the Far East and Africa during the correction of the nasal profile in these particular patients.

In these patients we find a very deep and flat nose profile that helps make their faces round and flat. It is possible to raise their nasal profile in order to let theface emerge, making it more visible and detailed.

The correction can be done by needle or cannula, but personally I prefer this second solution for the perfect uniformity on the profile and for the better safety profile that assures.

In the few pages that follow we can see some practical case studies from the pre-picture through the practical decisions during the procedure to the final result.

Example 1: A case treated with needle

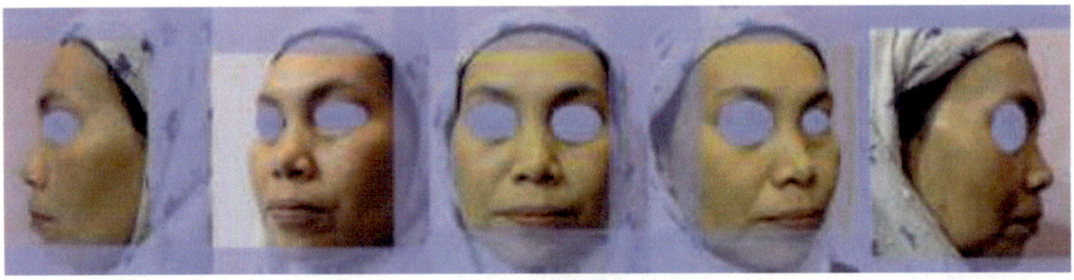

Figure 9. Patient study: 52 year old, Fitzpatrick photo-type 3-4. She is studied before the procedure during a medical course. The nasal profile is quite deep. There is also present an initial depression of the tears valley. I study the patient also in mimical phase and I do not see a particular mimical defect. So I decide to treat the nasal bridge with a middle reticulated absorbable filler. In this case, I use the technique with needle.

Anyway, normally, 0.2–0.3 ml of gel. Then I decide where to start the 1st injection for the nasal profile. Normally I inject from Rhinion to Nasion, deep on the bone. (c).

Immediately it is possible to see the bump caused by the injection of the gel. Gently, with the right hand, I proceed to the massage from up to down (e). During the injection, it is mandatory to keep the first and second fingers of the noninjecting hand on the sides of the nose, to avoid spreading of the gel in this area. I have seen many cases of migration of the gel also in the inferior eyelid. Pay a lot of attention to this in particular.

Immediately after, I proceed to the second injection just below the previous (f) always pushing the usual 2 fingers on the sides of the nose. I proceed then to the gently massage with both the right and left hands (g). Then I proceed to the final injection in the lower part of the nose to underline a little bit also the nasal tip (h). This is also a very fine passage. The compression of the nose, during the procedure (i). If the nose bleeds too little. immediately it becomes difficult to understand exactly the right correction. For this reason it is very important to avoid important ecchymosis of this area. I proceed to do a little correction also of the sides of the nose, between the alar great cartilage and the triangular (immediately above) to try to reduce nasal flaring (l-m).

In the preliminary study, I observed an important regression also of the chin. All the areas of the face are strictly connected to each other and a good aesthetic doctor must always have a three-dimensional approach. In so many Asian patients it is possible to see this little defect (2nd skeletal classes are so frequent). I inject for this reason at the Pogonion, down on the bone, 1 ml of Hyaluronic acid gel to get an improvement with a little protrusion of the chin (n).

http://dx.doi.org/10.5772/62066

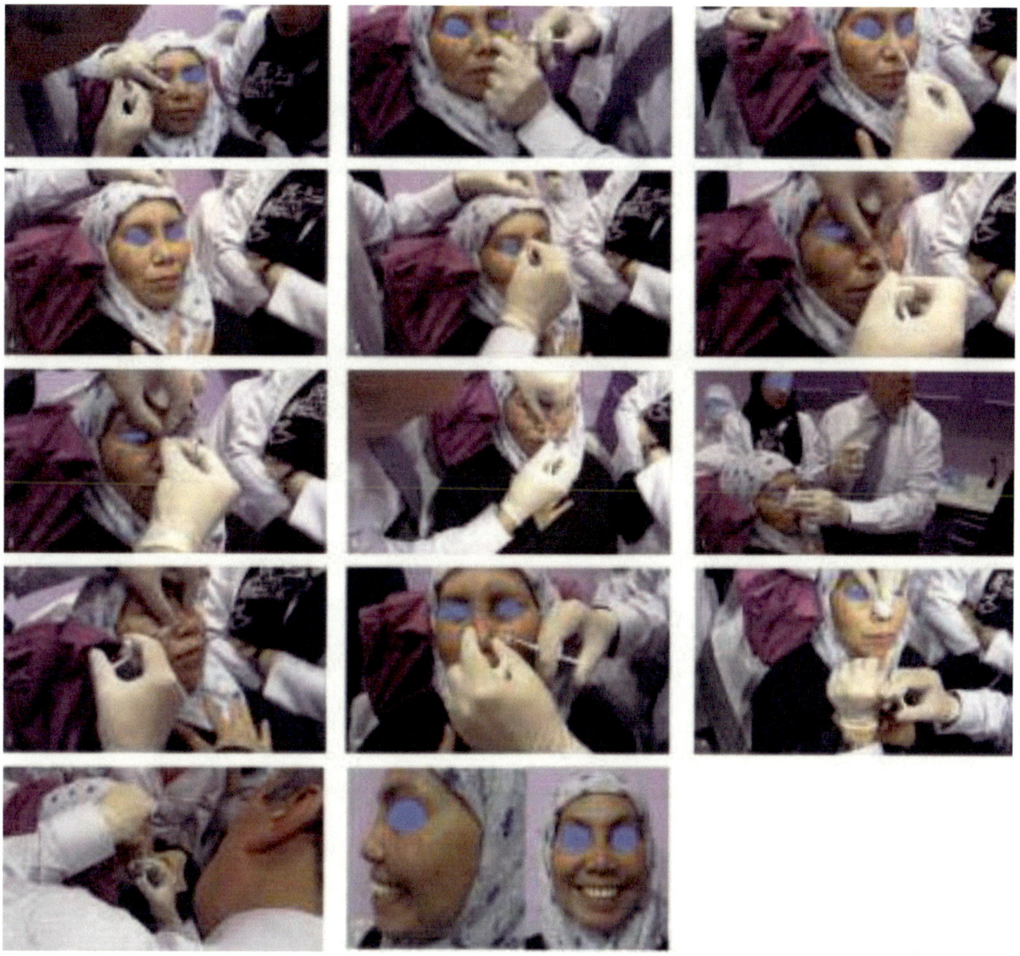

Figure 10. The procedure: I start the procedure in the malar-zygomatic area (a and b). I draw a line 1.3 cm under the orbital bone. I inject normally in 2 or 3 points, down on the bone. It is impossible to say exactly how much. Normally I say "not too much!!"

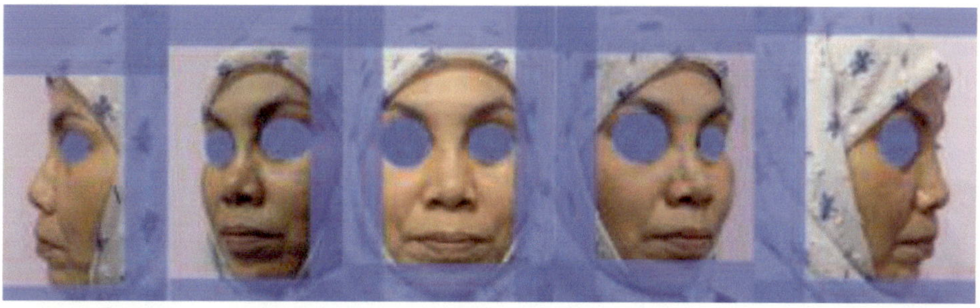

Figure 11. The results are immediate, as always while using a resorbable filler. They will last for many months, normally more than 1 year.

I finish the procedure with the correction of all the little defects that are is possible to see in the nasal bridge (o).

At the end, the correction must be perfect in all the projections of the nose.

The patient is studied also in mimical phase. The smile appears to be more balanced, visible in an important way, during movements (impossible to render just with some pictures) (p).

After 15 days it is a good rule to see the patients for a follow-up, to take pictures, but many times also for a little touchup, which in particular will allow you to have better and longer-lasting results.

Normally, patients come back after 1 year to make a new correction to maintain results.

The correction of nasal profile in Far Eastern and African patients can be made, of course, also with the cannula. I use as well the 25G cannula x 50 mm. Results are immediate and long-lasting.

All the passages are exactly the same as in all other patients. The suggestion, in this case, can be that of keeping the usual fingers of the noninjecting hand just near the sides of the cannula to obtain finally a narrow bridge that is more normally enjoyed by these patients.

7. Conclusions

The correction of nasal profile is a safe and easy technique. Results are immediate and long-lasting, more than in other facial areas.

The rules to obtain perfect results must be followed mainly to avoid side effects, which in this area can be unpleasant and also long-lasting. However, all possible side effects and especially skin necrosis heal well with time (2–3 months).

The perfect understanding of the genesis of the possible defects is the right way to use the right technique and finally have a good result.

It must become technical baggage of every aesthetic doctor.

Author details

Alessio Redaelli*

Address all correspondence to: mail@docredaelli.com

Visconti di Modrone Medical Center, Milan, Italy

http://dx.doi.org/10.5772/62066

References

[1] Redaelli A. Medical rhinoplasty with hyaluronic acid and botulinum toxin A: a very simple and quite effective technique. *J Cosm Dermatol*. 2008; 7, 210-220.

[2] Redaelli A, Braccini F. *The Medical Rhinoplasty: Basic Principles and Clinical Practice*. Firenze: OEO; 2010.

[3] Levignac J, Chalaye JC, Chalaye JM, Mahe E and Riu R. Morphology of the nose. Importance of the orificial mechanism. Surgical repercussions. *Ann Chir Plast Esthet*. 1986;31(4):309-318.

[4] Jasin ME. Nonsurgical rhinoplasty using dermal fillers. *Facial Plast Surg Clin N Am*. 2013; 21(2):241-252.

Chapter 14

Nonsurgical Rhinoplasty

Alexander Z. Rivkin

Additional information is available at the end of the chapter

http://dx.doi.org/10.5772/62065

Abstract

The goal of this chapter is to acquaint the experienced injector with the technique of Nonsurgical Rhinoplasty (NSR). This is an advanced technique and I am assuming that readers will be thoroughly familiar with how to perform cosmetic injections. I am also assuming that readers are knowledgeable about the various fillers and injectables available today in the United States.

NSR provides the first noninvasive alternative to surgical rhinoplasty, accomplishing the cosmetic goals of contour improvement without the risks and downtime of surgery. NSR is not a replacement for rhinoplasty and is appropriate in a specific subgroup of rhinoplasty candidates, which will be characterized. The procedure is currently being performed in a variety of ways, as described in the literature review. This chapter will detail the optimal methods of carrying out NSR based on a 10-year, 2500-patient experience with the technique. Discussion will also include critical safety concerns, tips on how to get the best results possible, and complication management. Being prepared for complications is a particular concern with NSR because timely intervention is so critical in cases of ischemic events. Patient selection, knowledge of the anatomy, meticulous technique, and a focus on safety is the key to success with this procedure. Overall, NSR is safe, precise, effective, and versatile. My patients are thrilled with their results, and I have made it the foundation of a thriving practice.

Keywords: Rhinoplasty, injection, nonsurgical, Artefill, methyl methacrylate, Radiesse, calcium hydroxylapatite, Voluma, hyaluronic acid, Restylane, Juvederm, nose job, necrosis, vascular embolism, ischemia, plastic surgery

1. Introduction

Surgical rhinoplasty remains one of the most popular cosmetic procedures performed on the face. Statistics from the American Academy of Facial Plastic Surgery and the American Society of Aesthetic Plastic Surgery put the number of rhinoplasties performed in the United States in

2012 at around 190,000 [1,2]. This number is relatively unchanged from what it was in 1997, prior to the FDA approval of cosmetic botulinum toxin and hyaluronic acid fillers. As with any surgical procedure, patients undergoing rhinoplasty are subject to significant risks, recovery time and expense. Until recently, patients who wanted to avoid surgery have never had a viable alternative procedure that could accomplish the cosmetic goals of rhinoplasty noninvasively. With the advent of long-lasting injectable fillers, however, physicians and patients have embraced a nonsurgical surrogate.

I first performed primary Nonsurgical Rhinoplasty (NSR) using calcium hydroxyapatite injectable filler in 2003, prior to the publication or report of such a procedure being done in the United States. The novelty of the procedure caught the attention of the media, and I performed it on several prominent national news programs and shows. This sparked the interest of the public and doctors around the country began to offer NSR to their patients. Several small studies have documented the safety and efficacy of the procedure since then [3,4,5]. Due to the simplicity and efficacy of NSR, it has steadily grown in popularity over the last decade. Since 2003, I have had the privilege to perform over 2500 of these procedures in my clinic, using a variety of injectable fillers, with great success.

2. History

The idea of injecting substances under the nasal skin to improve cosmesis is not new. Corning and Gersuny first described injecting liquid paraffin into the nose to correct saddle nose deformity at the beginning of the nineteenth century. The practice was quickly embraced but just as quickly abandoned because of the severe long-term adverse effects of paraffin [6]. In 1919, Bruning tried to correct postoperative cosmetic nasal imperfections with fat injection [7]. The technique was ultimately not very well accepted because the fat grafts showed poor survival duration [8]. In 1986, Webster presented a 20-year retrospective study of microdroplet silicone injection into the nasal bridge to correct postsurgical nasal defects [9]. The study reported mostly positive results, but many physicians, aware of horrific reports of complications from the 1960s and 1970s, have remained wary of silicone injections.

The first modern study of NSR was published by Han *et al.* in 2006 [10]. It was an 11-patient pilot study, looking at the safety and efficacy of dorsal augmentation NSR using hyaluronic acid (Restylane, Medicis, Scottsdale, Ariz.) mixed with autologous fibroblasts. Hyaluronic acid (HA) is a glycosaminoglycan that is a major component of connective, dermal, and neural tissue in most mammals. Cross-linked HA has been widely used as an injectable filler since it was FDA approved in 2003. Because of its biocompatibility, no allergy testing is required. The HA in Restylane is produced by bacterial fermentation. The authors injected an average of 0.8 cc into the nasal dorsum of their patients, overcorrecting by 20%. Of the 6 patients that Han *et.al* were able to get follow-up data on, there were no adverse events and the augmentation effect was still persisting at 12 months. Later that year, Beer published a case report where he successfully corrected a dorsal cosmetic defect with Restylane [11].

Also that year, *Laryngoscope* published a report by Nyte where he successfully injected calcium hydroxyapatite (CaHA, Radiesse, Merz, San Mateo, CA) to correct collapse of the internal nasal valve in 23 patients [12]. Radiesse is a suspension of 30% of CaHA microspheres, 25–45μm in size, in a mix of glycerin, carboxymethyl-cellulose, and water. It is fully biocompatible because CaHA is identical to the mineral portion of human bone and teeth [13]. Radiesse was first approved as a radiologic marker and for use in vocal fold augmentation. FDA approval for cosmetic use came in 2006. Nyte's technique of injecting through the inside of the nose seemed to show some cosmetic correction along with the functional improvement. This is, however, the only study that advocated intranasal injection.

Several papers emerged in the next year, including two small studies of Radiesse for cosmetic improvement of the nose. In the paper by Stupak *et al.*, the authors reported on a 13-patient prospective single-arm trial with blinded evaluators of before and after pictures [5]. They injected post-rhinoplasty patients seeking minor contour improvement. Areas injected included dorsum, supratip, nasal sidewall, and ala. Mean amount injected was 0.18cc. They did not inject the nasal tip due to concern that Radiesse would diffuse after injection and the tip would lose definition. There were no adverse events and patient satisfaction and evaluator ratings were good, but follow-up was only 2 months. Dayan *et al.* described their experience with Radiesse NSR in 8 patients over the span of 2 years [14]. The volume they used ranged from 0.3cc to 1.6cc and the corrections were mostly to the dorsum, radix, and supratip. Duration of effect was estimated to be around 1 year. They encountered no complications. At the end of their paper they made a point of mentioning that Dayan had performed revision rhinoplasty on a patient who had received Radiesse 14 months earlier without complication.

The other paper that year was by De LaCerda *et al.* from Brazil [15]. They presented a 2-patient experience with NSR using small amounts of porcine collagen on one patient (0.35 cc) and hyaluronic acid (Voluma, Allergan, Irvine, Calif.) on the other (0.20 cc); follow-up was 4 months and 1 year, respectively. Areas injected included the nasofrontal angle, nasolabial angle, the dorsum, and the tip.

In 2009, Humphrey and Dayan published a paper describing their preferences and techniques of NSR in 22 patients with HA and an unspecified number with CaHA [16]. They advocated using CaHA over HA because the latter absorbed water unpredictably. They considered injecting significant amounts of HA into virgin noses dangerous due to the risk of vascular compromise from the hydrophilic swelling of the product. They recommended injecting filler subdermally and avoiding the tip and supratip area. The only complications that they observed from the technique came after injecting HA into the tip area of two post-rhinoplasty patients, one by Dayan and one by an outside injector. These were both cases of ischemia. Dayan's patient was a mild case of Raynaud's-like phenomenon on the nasal tip and had no sequelae due to treatment with Hyaluronidase. The outside injector's case was a more serious case of ischemia that resolved with Nitropaste and Hyaluronidase. Although necrosis was avoided, they report that the patient developed aesthetically displeasing skin changes 1 year afterward. Notably, they again write that Dayan has had no trouble performing rhinoplasty on post-CaHA NSR patients. This is interesting because it contradicted numerous anecdotal accounts by other rhinoplasty surgeons at meetings and on the Internet that injectable fillers were causing catastrophic scarring and damage to the nasal tissues [17].

In 2010, we published our 4-year experience with CaHA NSR, comprising 385 patients [18]. We injected virgin noses as well as patients who had undergone rhinoplasty surgery in the past. We used volumes ranging from 0.3 cc to 0.5 cc of CaHA. We showed the procedure to be extremely safe. Two serious complications were encountered in patients who had undergone multiple revision rhinoplasties. They consisted of ischemia that progressed to small areas of tissue necrosis at the tip and ala despite treatment with Nitropaste and oral steroids. The rate of minor complications like cellulitis, prolonged swelling, or prolonged bruising was very low. Interestingly, a history of previous rhinoplasty surgery did not increase the risk of minor complications. The only exception was that post-rhinoplasty patients did have an increased incidence of prolonged erythema. We documented successful injection of all areas of the nose, including the tip, ala, dorsum, sidewall, and radix. We were surprised that the cosmetic effect of CaHA did not, on average, last as long as we expected. A significant number of patients showed evidence of resorption of the material as early as six months after injection.

In 2012, Kim and Ahn published a paper on a standardized NSR technique for Asian patients using mostly CaHA (except for tip injection, where they used HA) [19]. They reported their experience with 87 patients. Unlike most authors, they used 2% Xyocaine for anesthesia, injecting the infratrochlear and external nasal nerves as well as placing boluses at the nasal tip and the columnella-labial angle. Their technique consists of three steps. First, the columnella and columnella-labial angle is augmented with an injection from the tip down to the nasal spine. Second, the dorsum is augmented with a single injection, advancing the needle from the tip to the radix and injecting upon withdrawal, as in the first step. The third step involves shaping the tip with small, superficial bolus injections of HA. Four minor complications are reported, none of them ischemic. They end the paper with a series of sensible guidelines to avoid complications and achieve optimal cosmetic results.

In 2013, Kurkjian and Rohrich published their recommendations on technique for NSR [20]. The extent of their experience with the technique is not stated. They advocate low-pressure injection with HA fillers only, using the smallest possible needles. According to them, Sculptra and Radiesse should be avoided due to their irreversibility and the danger of long-term palpability under relatively thin nasal skin. For patients desiring permanent nonsurgical correction, permanent fillers should be avoided and fat should be used instead. They recommend using Restylane in all areas of the nose because it is relatively less hydrophilic. The exception is the tip, where Juvederm is also recommended, taking advantage of postinjection hydrophilic swelling for patients who want to increase tip fullness. In their experience, HA has much higher longevity in the nose, lasting up to 2–3 years in some areas (I have not seen evidence of this kind of duration in my HA NSR patients). They consider filler injection to be useful in the correction of post-rhinoplasty contour irregularities.

This year I published a prospective, blinded study on the safety and efficacy of injecting methyl methacrylate (Artefill, Suneva, Santa Barbara, CA) to correct nasal contour deficiencies [21]. Artefill is a third-generation methyl methacrylate filler in a collagen carrier that was FDA approved in 2006 for nasolabial fold correction. The filler is 20% methyl methacrylate and 80%

http://dx.doi.org/10.5772/62065

bovine collagen. Allergy testing for the carrier is commonly done 2 weeks prior to injection. The particles are smooth and 30–50 microns in size. I have been using Artefill off-label for NSR since 2006 with no complications in about 750 patients. In my experience, 3–5 injection sessions are necessary because the body quickly absorbs the collagen carrier and the methyl methacrylate stimulates fibroblast proliferation to a variable degree. For the study, I injected the product over 3 sessions, spaced 1 month apart. Results were evaluated by me, an independent, blinded MD evaluator, and the patient. With 1 year follow-up on 19 patients, we all observed excellent cosmetic effect and no complications of any kind. An example of the results we obtained is illustrated in Fig. 3.

3. Technique

NSR corrects mild or moderate cosmetic nasal irregularities. I perform this procedure to achieve the following cosmetic goals:

1. Raise and better define an underdeveloped nasal dorsum. This is most popular among my Asian patients.
2. Raise and better define a ptotic tip, as in Fig. 1.
3. Camouflage a dorsal bump. The dorsum is leveled by injecting filler above and below the bump, as in Fig. 2.
4. Correct asymmetry of the tip or dorsum by subtly augmenting the weaker side.
5. Correct post-rhinoplasty contour defects. Most commonly, these present as saddle nose deformity or other type of dorsal cartilage collapse, polly beak deformity, dorsal asymmetry due to asymmetric scarring, asymmetry of the tip due to postsurgical scarring or cartilage over-resection and alar foreshortening.

Injectors around the world have used a variety of materials to achieve the aesthetic recontouring of NSR. Currently, hyaluronic acid (HA) is the most popular filler material due to its reversibility (via injection of Hyaluronidase). There are a number of reports and editorials on technique in the literature. Most of these have been summarized above.

I consider HA, in its most common formulations of Juvederm and Restylane, to be the best material for the beginner or the occasional injector of the nose. The ability to dissolve HA is a critical safety feature for injectors who are not yet experts in the technique. Juvederm and Restylane are effective for basic NSR goals, such as augmenting the bridge and camouflaging minor dorsal bumps. These fillers struggle to perform, however, in the more advanced applications of this technique. Juvederm and Restylane are relatively soft materials. They can only provide moderate augmentation of the dorsum, they cannot lift a drooping tip very much and they are poor at sculpting defining points of the tip and the sidewall of the nose. In my experience, these HA fillers last an average of 6–8 months.

Perlane is a formulation of HA that is an improvement over Juvederm and Restylane for NSR. Its increased density permits the advanced injector to sculpt more effectively. It has less of a

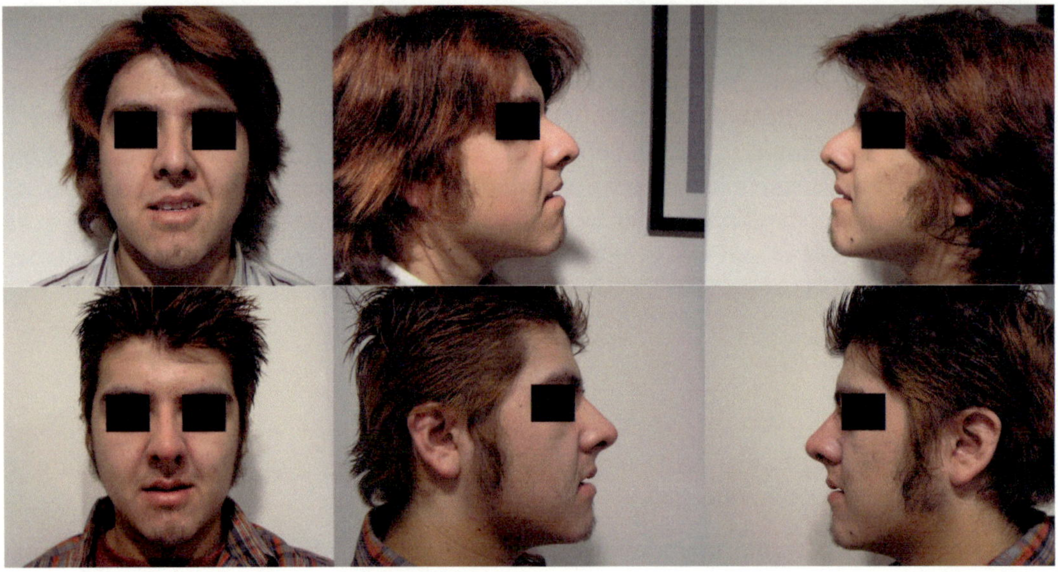

Figure 1. CaHA NSR to lift a ptotic nasal tip and augment the nasal radix. The "Before" pictures are on top, "After" on the bottom. The net result is a straighter nose on profile that appears smaller because it blends better into the rest of the face.

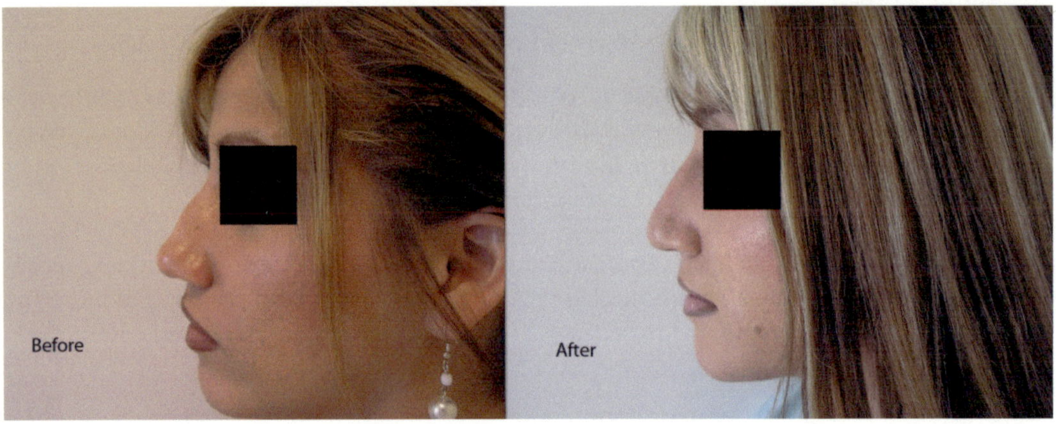

Figure 2. HA NSR to camouflage a dorsal hump. The patient wanted to use a minimum of product to make her profile straighter. She believed a slight curve would make her nose look more natural.

tendency to spread, so better definition can be achieved. Perlane also lasts somewhat longer in the nose than Juvederm and Perlane – about 8 months in my experience. Prior to the FDA approval of Voluma, I used Perlane for patients who wanted the added safety of a reversible filler.

I have used calcium hydroxyapatite (CaHA – Radiesse, MERZ Aesthetics Inc., San Mateo, CA) in most of my NSR procedures. Radiesse received FDA approval in 2006 for correcting

http://dx.doi.org/10.5772/62065

moderate to severe wrinkles and HIV-related facial volume changes. Prior to that it was approved for vocal cord augmentation and I was using it off-label in the nose. As a non-HA filler, CaHA is not reversible. Hypersensitivity reactions to CaHA are extremely uncommon and reports of other adverse events do not differ significantly from reports for HA fillers. Side effects noted of CaHA include:

- Nodules (generally associated with lip augmentation or injection in areas with little subdermal space, e.g., infraorbital area) (Smith, 2007) (Tzikas, 2008)
- Granulomas (Lee MJ, 2008)
- Skin necrosis (Dayan SH and Arkins JP, 2011)
- Redness, erythema, and swelling (Siclovan, 2009)

The advantages of CaHA are its relative persistence of effect (average of 9–10 months in my experience, but quite variable between 6 and 12 months) and its high density. This last quality allowed me to effectively sculpt noses to my patients' satisfaction. It is possible to significantly elevate a droopy tip without excessive rounding. In fact, CaHA makes it possible to precisely create aesthetically pleasing tip defining points in patients with rounded and poorly defined tips. CaHA also makes it possible to significantly raise and add real definition to an underdeveloped dorsum – a quality that my Asian patients particularly appreciate.

With the FDA approval of Voluma in October of 2013, injectors gained a valuable new tool that seems to confer longer duration of effect than any other filler. Voluma is more cross-linked than other HA fillers and has a higher percentage of low molecular weight hyaluronic acid, making it exceptionally smooth, viscous, and cohesive. Increased cross-linking makes the filler more resistant to enzymatic degradation. Under study conditions, duration of effect was up to 2 years [22], but anecdotal reports from the investigators indicate the filler to be even longer lasting than that. Because of the duration of effect and its reversibility, I have been using Voluma for the majority of my NSR cases over the last 5 months. It performs well for the most part, but I find that in patients that need extensive elevation of their tip or dorsum, Radiesse is still the only filler thick enough to provide the desired lift. In these patients, my NSR combines Voluma and Radiesse.

I perform this procedure with the patient sitting up straight in the chair, as in Fig. 5. After taking standardized photographs, I use a compounded triple anesthetic cream for 15–20 min prior to the procedure (the materials I use are pictured in Fig. 4). My assistant will remove the cream and the patient will ice the area to be injected. During the injection, my assistant taps the patient's contralateral shoulder to distract their attention from the injection. I have found that alcohol works fine to clean the area and prevent infections. I prefer a thin-walled 29 gage half-inch needle when using any of the fillers – Voluma, Radiesse, or Artefill. If that is not available, I use a thin-walled 28 gage one-inch needle. I perform injections for the most part as shallow linear threads, placing small amounts of filler as I withdraw the needle. I will place filler into the area of the radix, dorsum, sidewall, tip, columnella, and ala as needed to correct each individual irregularity. I will then massage and mold the filler to blend into the desired contour. The patient goes home with instructions to avoid alcohol and strenuous exercise that

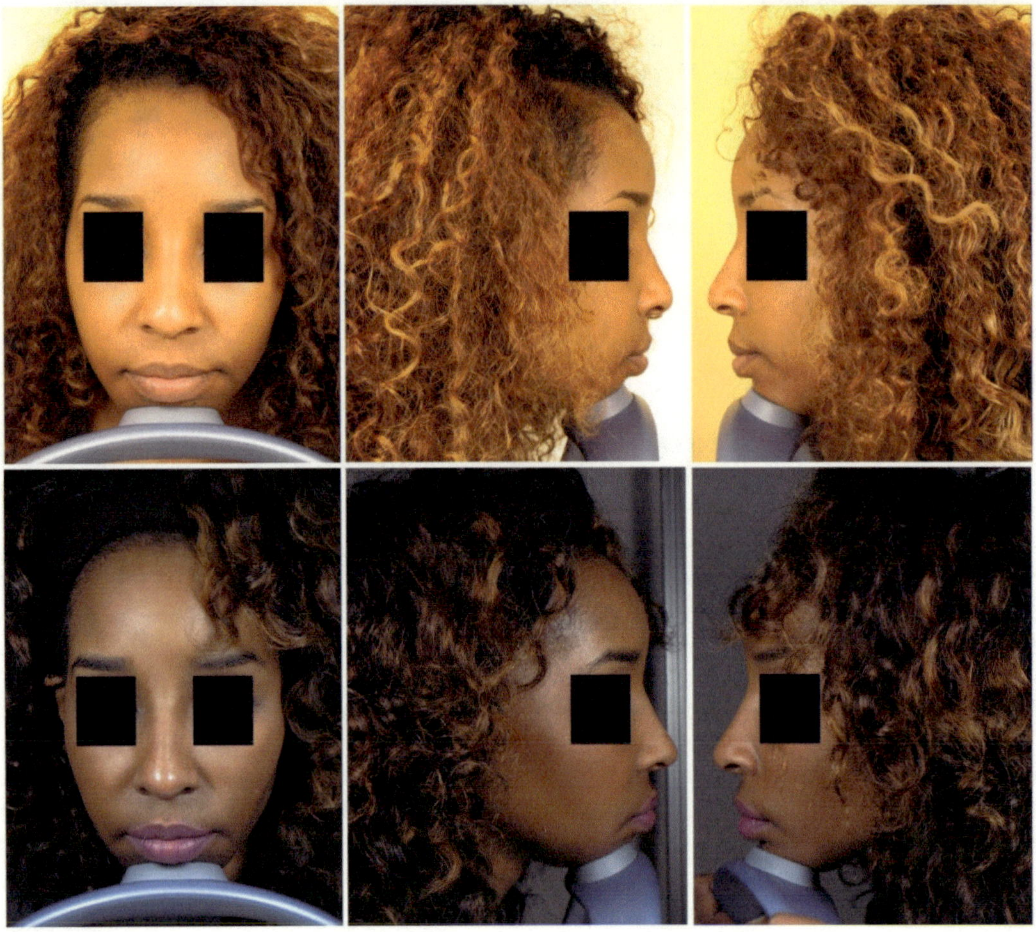

Figure 3. Artefill NSR to refine and straighten the dorsum and tip from both the profile and straight on views. This patient wanted to have a thinner appearing nose from the frontal view and a straighter and more refined looking dorsum and tip from the profile.

day, as well as heavy sunglasses for two weeks. I agree with Kim and Ahn's observation that the volume effect of most fillers decreases by about 25% within the first month or two [19]. For this reason, my procedure includes a complementary follow-up visit 3 weeks after the initial injection, where I can touch-up the results.

In my experience, there are several types of patients that seek NSR. Most commonly, it is the younger patient who cannot afford the time or resources required for postsurgical recovery. They hear about the procedure through friends and the Internet. They mostly present with mild or moderate cosmetic irregularities. Having studied the before and after pictures and read about the procedure, they understand that it is not a technique that can physically reduce the size of the nose, so I rarely see patients with severely large noses.

http://dx.doi.org/10.5772/62065

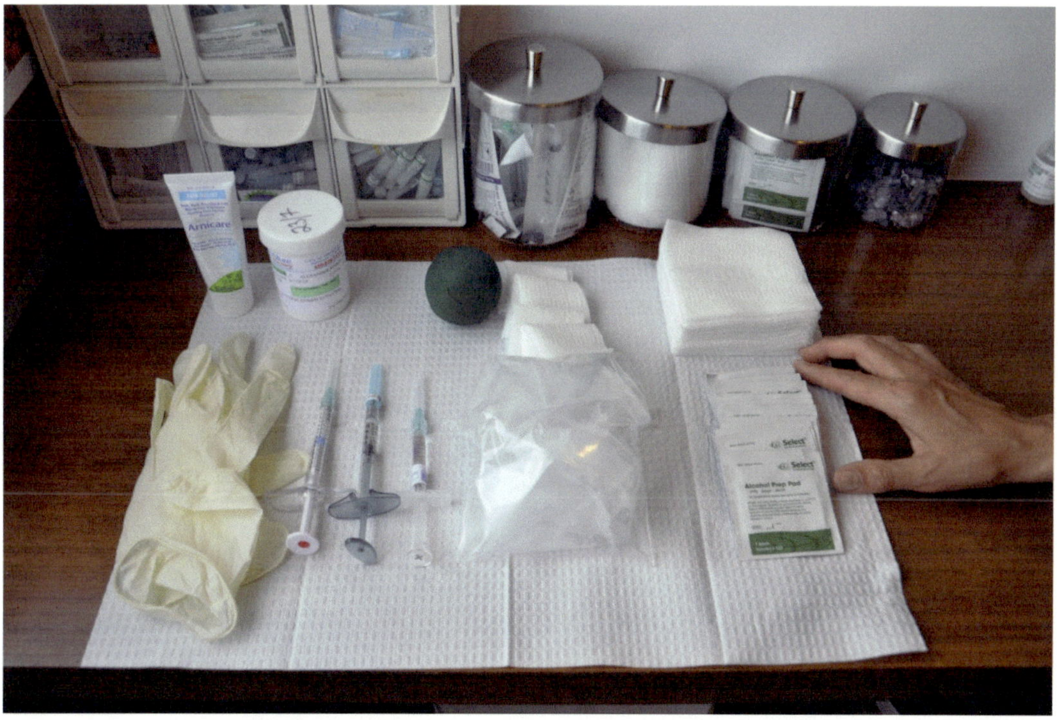

Figure 4. Equipment necessary for NSR. Radiesse, Voluma, and Perlane are all displayed with the first two as presplit half syringes (using a Luer-Lock connector and a 1cc syringe). I try to use the smallest possible needle gage – 27 or 28 G thin-walled needles are my preference. The photograph displays the four main methods of pain control in my injectables practice. Topical numbing cream is a compounded 23% Lidocaine, 7% Tetracaine mixture. Ice and a stress ball are important, but most important is my assistant's hand, which distracts the patient by tapping on the shoulder opposite to where I am standing.

About a third of my NSR patients are Asian, as in Fig. 6. These patients commonly desire an increase in the height and definition of their dorsum and radix, as well as improvement in the definition and projection of their nasal tip. These patients are usually young and cannot afford surgery. They are also often wary of unnatural surgical results, describing people with visible or overly large dorsal grafts that they have seen in the Asian community. Like many patients who opt for this procedure, they want to see the cosmetic change they desire, but only if their nose retains a natural appearance and no one can tell that they have had an aesthetic procedure.

Both of these kinds of patients usually choose the temporary procedure using a CaHA filler like Radiesse or an HA filler like Perlane or Voluma. They are aware that I commonly use Artefill for long-lasting to permanent results but want to try out the effect before they commit. Once the effect fades, some of these patients decide to continue with the temporary filler but many switch over to Artefill.

Another common category of patients presenting for this procedure are the ones who have desired cosmetic improvement in their nose for a long time, but have been afraid of surgical

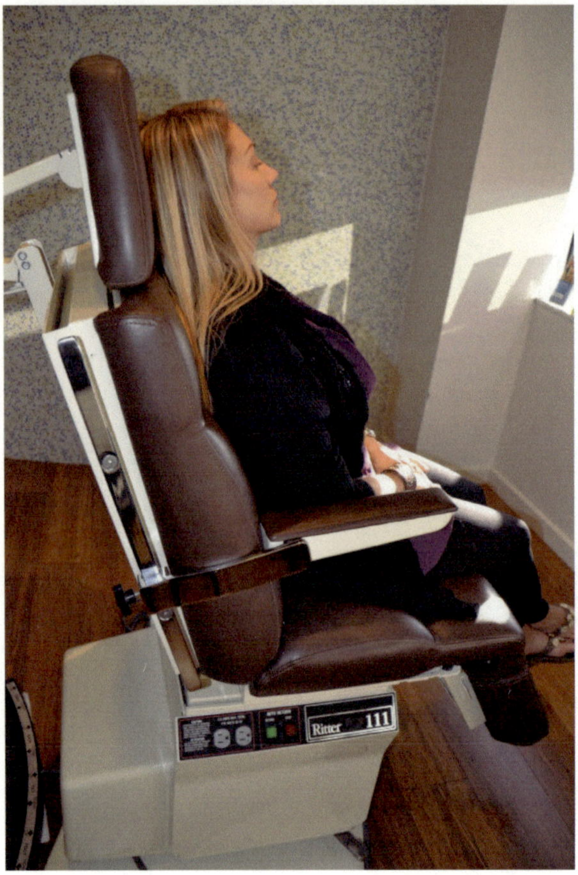

Figure 5. Correct patient position for NSR. She is relaxed and sitting comfortably with her head resting on the back of the chair. Movement is minimized. There is no tissue redistribution, as there would be if the patient was lying flat, so cosmetic results are optimally accurate.

and anesthesia risks. These patients present with a variety of aesthetic complaints. Most are appropriate for the NSR technique, but some require reduction and have to be turned away.

An important subset of the above patient group is those who consider their aesthetic complaint to be too minor to undergo surgical correction. They are bothered by their small bump or mild asymmetry but feel that surgery exacts too high of a price (both financial and temporal). These patients are mostly ideal candidates for NSR. A small amount of contour correction to restore symmetry or camouflage a small bump makes them very happy.

About a quarter of my patients have already had one or more surgical rhinoplasties. These patients present with a variety of aesthetic complaints, but all of them are disappointed in the aesthetic result of their surgery (or surgeries) and desire an effective alternative. Some opt for temporary fillers, but many choose methyl methacrylate so that they can "get it over with." Figure 7 illustrates one of those patients. Anyone who performs NSR must be aware that these patients present with technically challenging problems. Postsurgical scarring stiffens the skin

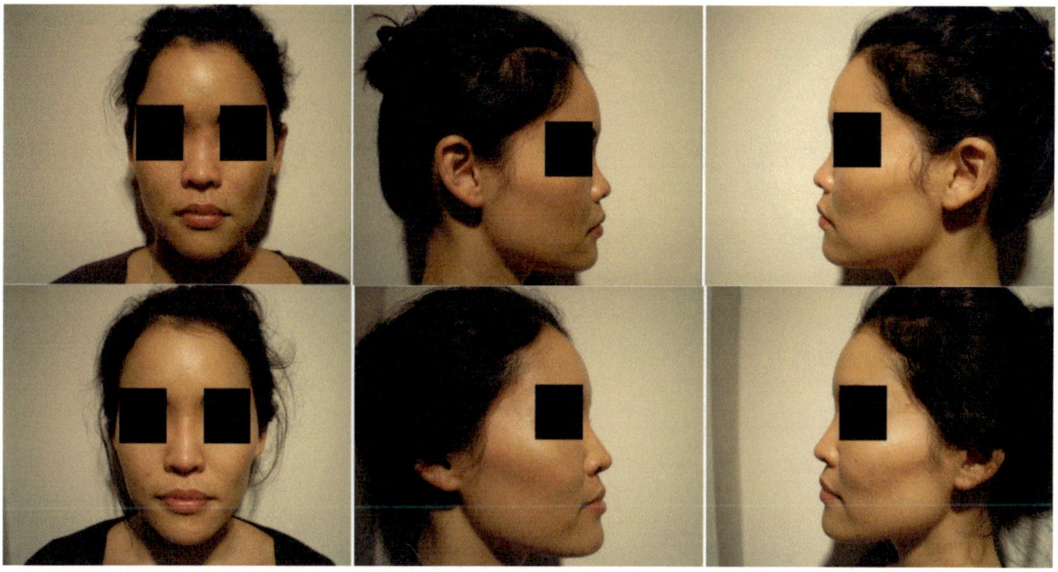

Figure 6. CaHA NSR to augment and better define a nasal bridge and tip in an Asian patient.

and limits the lift that can be achieved with filler injection. Injectors need to take care not to over-promise these patients. Their results are going to be, for the most part, relatively subtle. Most importantly, postsurgical skin has a more tenuous blood supply, especially around the tip and ala. The risk of ischemia and necrosis are significantly increased in these patients. Only the most experienced injectors should be treating them, since the complications of necrosis can be catastrophic.

Complications of NSR are relatively rare. This is not surprising, since the overall major complication rate for filler injections has been estimated to be less than one hundredth of one percent [4]. As described above, published studies are meager and mostly small, but they report few serious adverse events. Bruising, transient erythema, and short-term swelling represents most of the issues documented. The exceptions are the disturbing case reports that detail blindness and major necrosis of nasal tissue [5,6,7]. Since the doctors treating the complications and not those who injected the patients write most of these reports, conclusions about needle type, injection technique, and even material used are often difficult. Of the reports published by the actual injectors, we know that sudden pain, blanching, duskiness, and ecchymosis in the area being injected are all danger signals for ischemia and necrosis. Compromise of the blood supply to the skin in cases of filler injection can be caused by either intravascular embolism or small vessel compression by the filler.

Opthalmalgia and visual loss within minutes are signs of retinal artery embolism. Other signs of ophthalmic vasculature embolism include immediate diaphoresis, nausea, headache, opthalmoplegia, and ptosis [4].

In my experience, these complications can best be avoided by understanding the anatomy, always practicing safe injection technique, and having well-prepared protocols ready to launch

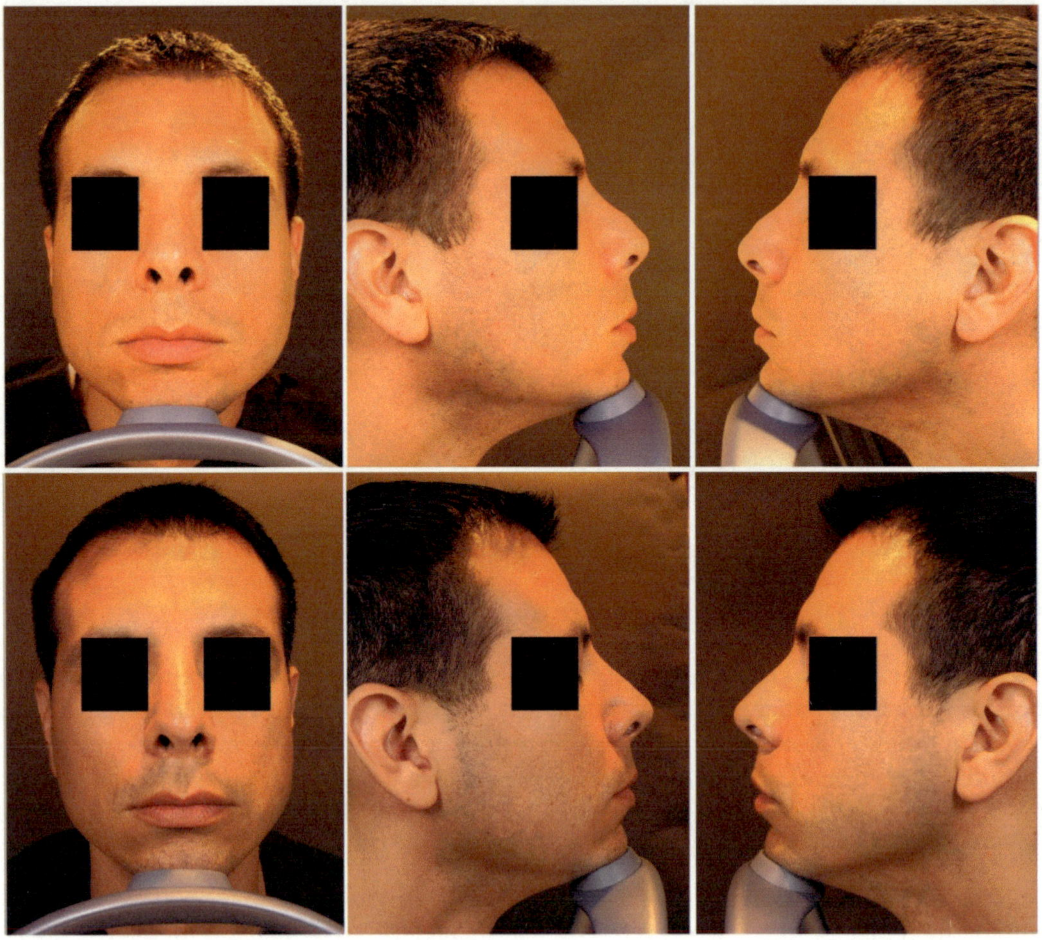

Figure 7. Artefill NSR to correct postsurgical contour irregularities and asymmetry of the dorsum and to lift the nasal tip. Lower series are 1 year after the last of three sessions of Artefill injections.

at any sign of danger. Our traditional understanding of the vascular anatomy of the external nose is illustrated in Fig 8.

A good injector is especially careful when injecting the radix and nasal sidewall, to avoid the dorsal nasal and angular branches, respectively. Based on Fig. 8, keeping one's injection points in the midline seems to ensure safety. This is surely true to some degree, but a recent paper by Saban *et al.* proposes that the external nasal vasculature is more interconnected than we think [23]. Using cadaver dissection and ultrasonography study of live subjects, the authors conclude that anastomoses between the internal and external carotid vascular systems are plentiful in the external nose. This plexus of vessels is located in the SMAS layer. Safe injection technique should therefore focus on keeping the needle deep instead of trying to avoid specific vessels.

http://dx.doi.org/10.5772/62065

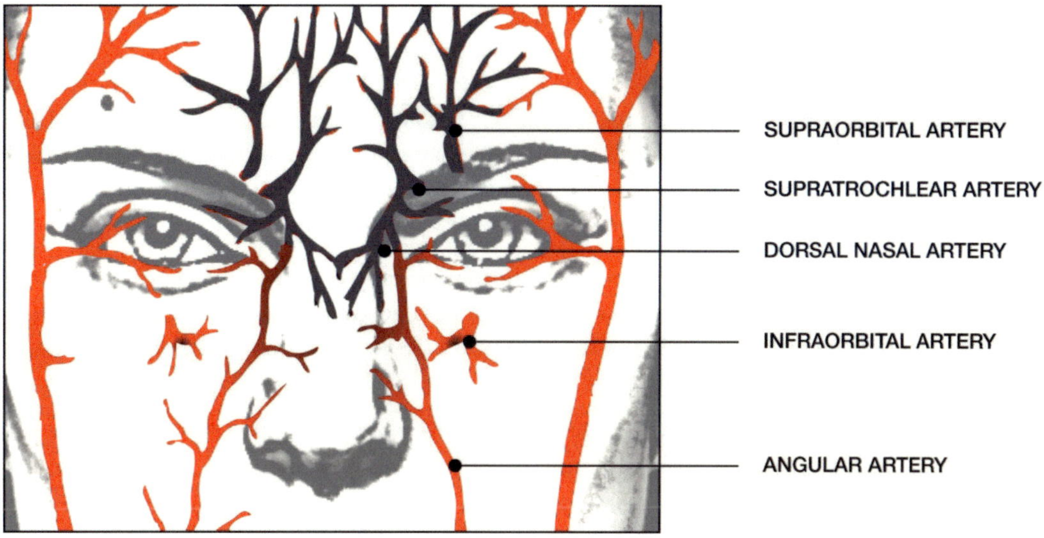

Figure 8. External arterial anatomy of the nose. Vessels originating from the External Carotid are in red, whereas those in black come from the Internal Carotid via the Opthalmic Artery.

Some clinicians have recommended aspiration prior to injection of filler in order to avoid vascular embolism. In my experience, this is a cumbersome practice with questionable benefits. Most fillers are thick gels. Building up enough negative pressure for aspiration of blood takes a lot of hand force and would only work for Voluma due to its smooth viscoelastic properties. Even in experienced hands, by the time one aspirates and then injects, the needle is no longer in the same place, rendering the test useless.

Rather than aspirating, I think that following accepted best practice standards for injecting filler is a more reliable way of preventing complications [8,9]:

1. Needles should be as small as possible so that filler flow rate is low.

2. Fillers should always be injected slowly and under low pressure, especially in the nasal area. The blindness complications in the literature occurred because a filler embolus was injected with enough force to overcome systolic blood pressure and travel up into the ophthalmic vasculature. Gentle injection technique should prevent this complication.

3. The needle should be advanced through the skin slowly and filler should only be flowing when the needle is moving out of the skin. This way, even if the tip of the needle is inside the lumen of a vessel at some point, only a tiny amount of filler will enter the vessel, as the needle will be out in the next moment.

4. Small volumes of filler should be introduced with each injection.

5. We always ice prior to injection. Ice decreases pain and shrinks blood vessels, making them less likely to be punctured.

Some authors advocate blunt tipped cannulas for all filler injection as a way to reduce complications and discomfort [10,11]. I think this is not a good idea in the nose. The weakness of cannulas is precision. It is much easier to know the exact location of a needle tip than the tip of a cannula that bends easily as it is advanced through the tissue. The aesthetics of the nose are particularly sensitive to the smallest contour asymmetries. One millimeter of fullness difference between two sides of the tip is clearly noticeable. One-millimeter deviation from the midline, when augmenting a dorsum, makes the nose appear off-center.

The literature contains reports of severe complications from every type of filler available, and I have successfully used a variety of materials in the nose. I do not believe that there is a material contraindicated for nasal injection. It is the skill and knowledge of the injector that is paramount to the success of the procedure.

While not really a complication, vaso-vagal episodes can be disturbing to the novice injector. Diaphoresis, sudden pallor, a sensation of nausea are all warning signs of an impending episode. It is more likely to happen if the patient has not eaten much prior to their appointment. In the setting of cosmetic injections, patients become vaso-vagal primarily because they are holding their breath in anticipation of pain. The frequency of these episodes dropped dramatically once we began to routinely remind our patients to breathe. Distraction shoulder tapping also helps them tolerate the injections without excessive anxiety. If the patient does become vaso-vagal, our routine is to immediately place them in reverse Trendelenberg position, increasing blood flow to the brain. We place an ice bag behind their neck and give them something sweet to drink like orange juice or Coke. We monitor their pulse and blood pressure manually. Most patients will recover fully within a few minutes. We have not yet had to use smelling salts.

Complication management starts with the preventative measures outlined above. If, however, the clinician suspects that an ischemic event is unfolding, there are immediate steps that he or she should be ready to take. First, injection should stop immediately. The area should be massaged vigorously in an effort to restore blood flow and Hyaluronidase should be injected into the area. A dose of 50–80 units should be sufficient. Even if a non-hyaluronic acid filler has been used, Hyaluronidase is useful because it dissolves some native hyaluronic acid and decreases interstitial pressure, easing blood flow. Topical 2% Nitroglycerin paste (Nitro-bid. Savage Labs, Melville NY) should be in the room and readily available to anyone performing this procedure. It is a great vasodilator that acts very quickly. In situations of potential ischemia, a small amount should be applied to the area in question and it should stay on for at least 15 min. The patient should take aspirin 325 mg immediately. If the skin becomes pink again and remains so after a period of observation of 15 min or so, I would feel comfortable sending the patient home on aspirin every 4 h for a day, warm compresses, and periodic massage of the area. If the skin becomes dusky, I would reapply the Nitropaste for another 30 min and consider reinjecting the area with Hyaluronidase. I would observe the patient in the office for the next hour or so, applying warm compresses and massaging the area. At this point, the patient should begin oral steroid therapy and oral antibiotics. I would give them a Medrol dose pack and make sure that they take the first dose right away. At this point, the patient should be seen in the office on a daily basis to monitor the progression of tissue damage. If

http://dx.doi.org/10.5772/62065

damage continues to unfold, the injector should consider hyperbaric oxygen therapy and referral to a plastic surgeon. My in-room safety kit, a.k.a. injectables "crash cart" is illustrated in Fig. 9.

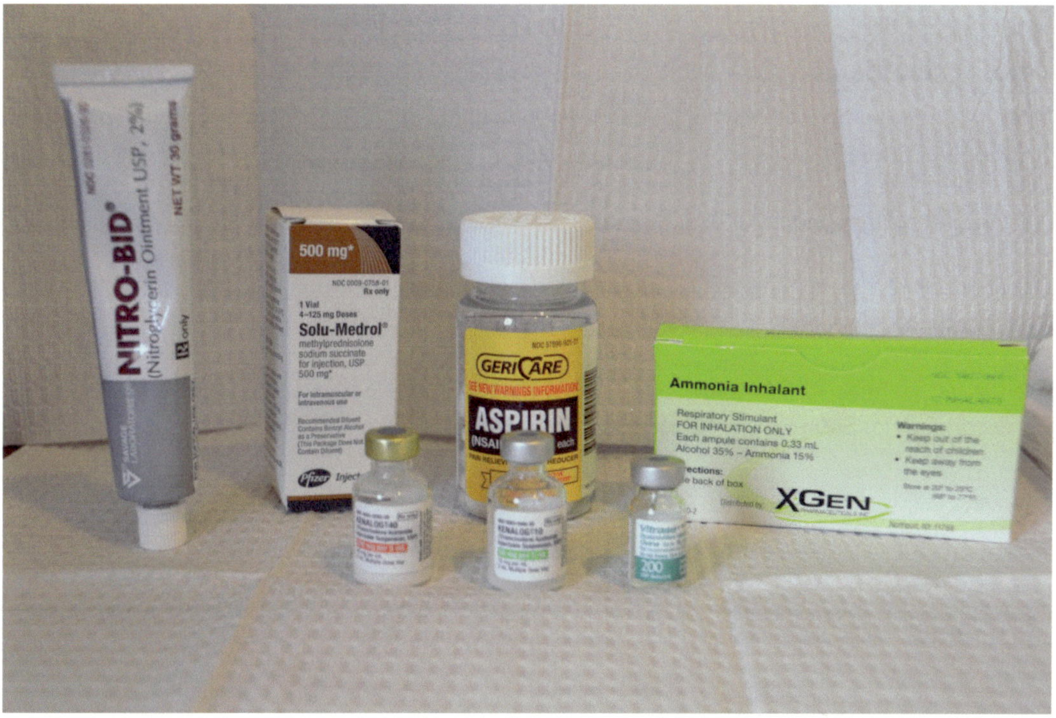

Figure 9. My in-room safety kit. Pictured are Hyaluronidase, Nitopaste, Aspirin, Kenalog, Solu-medrol, and smelling salts. These are the medications important to have on hand in every room.

When performed safely and correctly by an experienced and well-trained injector, NSR is a procedure that yields excellent patient satisfaction. It is not a replacement to rhinoplasty for all patients and I continue to refer those that are not candidates (mostly patients who need significant reduction) to my surgical colleagues. This procedure does, however, provide a valuable alternative to traditional surgery. It increases the pool of people wanting cosmetic correction of the nose, bringing in a significant population of patients who would never do surgery. In fact, recalling the statistics from AAFPRS and ASAPS, over the last 10 years that this procedure has become popular, it has not cut into the number of patients receiving surgical rhinoplasty [1,2]. For the patients who are candidates, it saves them expense, risk, and downtime. Finally, the precision of filler injection means that this procedure is in some cases superior to surgery in accomplishing patients' cosmetic goals. I have built a large practice upon this procedure and continue to receive many referrals from happy patients.

Acknowledgements

The author would like to thank Mimi Lam for her assistance with the layout and proofreading of this chapter.

Author details

Alexander Z. Rivkin

Address all correspondence to: arivkin@westsideaestehtics.com

Department of Dermatology, Division of Medicine, David Geffen, UCLA School of Medicine, Westside Aesthetics, Los Angeles, CA, USA

Conflict of interest: The author is on advisory boards and educational faculty for Allergan, Galderma, Merz, Solta Pharmaceuticals.

References

[1] http://www.aafprs.org/wp-content/themes/aafprs/pdf/AAFPRS-2012-REPORT.pdf

[2] http://www.plasticsurgery.org/Documents/news-resources/statistics/2012-Plastic-Surgery-Statistics/full-plastic-surgery-statistics-report.pdf

[3] Jacovella PF. Aesthetic nasal corrections with hydroxylapatite facial filler. Plast Reconstr Surg. 2008 May;121(5):338e-339e.

[4] Rokhsar C, Ciocon DH. Nonsurgical rhinoplasty: an evaluation of injectable calcium hydroxylapatite filler for nasal contouring. Dermatol Surg. 2008 Jul;34(7):944-6

[5] Stupak HD, Moulthrop TH, Wheatley P, Tauman AV, Johnson CM Jr. Calcium hydroxylapatite gel (Radiesse) injection for the correction of postrhinoplasty contour deficiencies and asymmetries. Arch Facial Plast Surg. 2007 Mar-Apr;9(2):130-6.

[6] Glicenstein J. The first "fillers," vaseline and paraffin From miracle to disaster. Ann Chir Plast Esthet 2007;52:157–61.

[7] Bruning P. Contribution a l'etude des greffes adipeuses. Bull Acad R Med Belg. 1919;28:440.

[8] Peer LA. Loss of weight and volume in human fat grafts. Plast Reconstr Surg. 1950;5:217.

[9] Webster RC, Hamdan US, Gaunt JM, Fuleihan NS, Smith RC. Rhinoplastic revisions with injectable silicone. Arch Otolaryngol Head Neck Surg. 1986;112: 269-276.

[10] Han SK, Shin SH, Kang HJ, Kim WK. Augmentation rhinoplasty using injectable tissue-engineered soft tissue: a pilot study. Ann Plast Surg. 2006 Mar;56(3):251-5.

[11] Beer KR. Nasal reconstruction using 20 mg/ml cross-linked hyaluronic acid. J Drugs Dermatol. 2006 May;5(5):465-6.

[12] Nyte CP. Spreader graft injection with calcium hydroxylapatite: a nonsurgical technique for internal nasal valve collapse. Laryngoscope. 2006 Jul;116(7):1291-2.

[13] Graivier MH, Bass LS, Busso M, Jasin ME, Narins RS, Tzikas TL. Calcium hydroxylapatite (Radiesse) for correction of the mid- and lower face: consensus recommendations. Plast Reconstr Surg. 2007 Nov;120(6 Suppl):55S-66S.

[14] Dayan SH, Greene RM, Chambers AA. Long-lasting injectable implant* for correcting cosmetic nasal deformities. Ear Nose Throat J. 2007 Jan;86(1):25-6.

[15] de Lacerda DA, Zancanaro P. Filler rhinoplasty. Dermatol Surg. 2007 Dec;33 Suppl 2:S207-12.

[16] Humphrey CD, Arkins JP, Dayan SH. Soft tissue fillers in the nose. Aesthet Surg J. 2009 Nov-Dec;29(6):477-84.

[17] http://deantoriumi.com/issue1-1.asp

[18] Rivkin A, Soliemanzadeh P. Nonsurgical Injection Rhinoplasty With Calcium Hydroxylapatite in a Carrier Gel (Radiesse): A 4-Year, Retrospective, Clinical Review. Cosmetic Dermatology. 2009 Dec;Vol. 22 No. 12: 619-624.

[19] Kim P, Ahn JT. Structured nonsurgical Asian rhinoplasty. Aesthetic Plast Surg. 2012 Jun;36(3):698-703.

[20] Kurkjian TJ, Ahmad J, Rohrich RJ. Soft-tissue fillers in rhinoplasty. Plast Reconstr Surg. 2014 Feb;133(2):121e-6e.

[21] Rivkin A. A prospective study of non-surgical primary rhinoplasty using a polymethylmethacrylate injectable implant. Dermatol Surg. 2014 Mar;40(3):305-13

[22] Jones D, Murphy DK. Volumizing hyaluronic Acid filler for midface volume deficit: 2-year results from a pivotal single-blind randomized controlled study. Dermatol Surg. 2013 Nov;39(11):1602-12.

[23] Saban Y, Andretto Amodeo C, Bouaziz D, Polselli R. Nasal arterial vasculature: medical and surgical applications. Arch Facial Plast Surg. 2012 Nov;14(6):429-36.